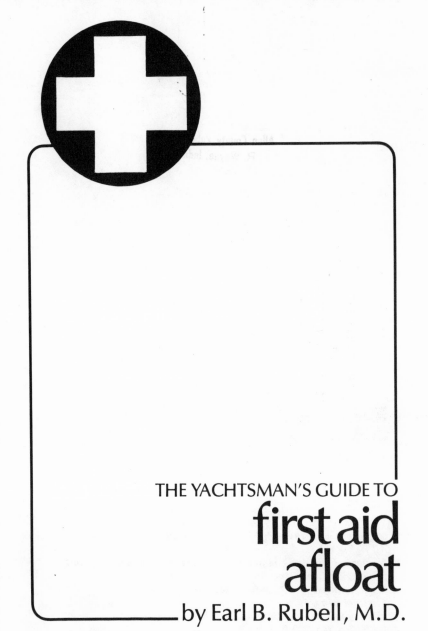

THE YACHTSMAN'S GUIDE TO
first aid
afloat
by Earl B. Rubell, M.D.

YACHTING/BOATING BOOKS • Ziff-Davis Publishing Co.
New York

Copyright © 1979 by Ziff-Davis Publishing Co.
All rights reserved.
No part of this book may be reproduced in any form without
permission in writing from the publisher.
Manufactured in the United States of America.
First printing, 1979.
Library of Congress Catalog Card Number 79–67632.
ISBN: 0–87165–033–9
Ziff-Davis Publishing Company
One Park Avenue
New York, N.Y. 10016

To those free spirits who venture out
onto great oceans in small boats this
book is dedicated as a toast:

"TO YOUR HEALTH"

Contents

Acknowledgments

Many colleagues have been very generous with their time and experience during the preparation of this guide. My deepest appreciation goes to: Mavis Burkhardt, R.N.; Benjamin Kagan, M.D.; Miriam Masse, R. Ph.; Alan Rosenberg, M.D.; Elliott Rosenberg, M.D.; Sheldon Rosenthal, M.D.; Leonard Skaist, M.D.; Lesther Winkler, M.D.

My thanks are also due to the library staff of the Cedars/Sinai Medical Center of Los Angeles and to the volunteers at the Poison Information Center, Children's Hospital of Los Angeles.

Getting Ready to Sail

You're going to sea. Whether for a day sail, a short cruise to a favorite local anchorage, or an extended voyage, you are looking forward to a relaxed, trouble-free journey marked by fair winds, sunny skies, and exuberant feelings. At the same time, you are aware that things sometimes go wrong. A crew member may fall overboard, equipment break, weather go foul, or someone become sick or injured. To ready yourself for these possibilities you carry appropriate spare parts and rehearse potential emergency procedures.

This volume is intenged to help you plan for and deal with medical problems which may arise. Preparation should include requiring each crew member to provide a written list of personal medical problems, medications taken, allergies to medication and potential problems and their treatment. Most of the subjects covered are applicable to the local boater, while much of the material is intended for use by long-distance sailors far removed from professional medical care.

It is important to remember that some of the suggestions to be made go beyond the usual advice to the layman. They may not always be the ideal medical care but they represent what I consider to be the best available alternative for the sick or injured sailor who cannot, because of distance or lack of communication, receive professional medical advaice or attention for a prolonged period of time after emergency first aid has been rendered.

How to Use This Guide

There are three sections for easy reference.

Section I: The Emergency Game Plan
An emergency is an unforeseen combination of circumstances requiring immediate action. A medical emergency is a frequent cause of panic, and panic rarely results in constructive action. It is easier to cope when you have given some thought beforehand as to what you will do if a given situation comes up. If you have fixed in mind an orderly sequence for evaluating an emergency, you will be able to establish priorities and take appropriate corrective measures. The first section presents a scheme for rapidly organizing the approach to a medical emergency.

Section II: Specific Problems and Suggested Solutions
A variety of illnesses and injuries, major and minor, urgent and routine, is presented. The subjects are arranged alphabetically. Each discussion presents briefly the nature of the problem, the identification of the need for treatment, and a systematic plan for giving aid.

Section III: The Medical Kit
This section describes the requirements for both short- and long-range cruising in terms of what to take, how it is used, appropriate dosages, and a scheme for organizing the contents of the kit for quick access.

Limitations

Before you begin to use this book, there are a few important things to understand in order for you to keep your role in perspective. Remember that there are limits to your ability to solve any problem, limits to your knowledge, to your experience, to the facilities and equipment available to you, and to your physical stamina. There may be a time when you must abandon one crisis to deal with another, which is more pressing. When the possible loss of a life is involved the decision can be very hard, and it is unfortunately of little use to a victim if the potential rescuer also perishes.

Finally, there are limits to the ability of the sick or injured body to heal itself. Despite your best efforts the outcome may not be what you desire. Fortunately, catastrophes are rare, and nature, with a little judicious assistance, tries to cure more often than not.

Section I
The Emergency
Game Plan

When a medical emergency arises there frequently seem to be many things which need to be done immediately. A disorganized attempt to do them all at once frequently results in failure to accomplish anything. It is essential to identify problems quickly and to place them in order of importance. A good way to do this is to ask yourself a series of questions. Assume only one person is available to give aid. Obviously, with more help responsibilities can be divided and more than one problem dealt with at the same time. In presenting the game plan I will not describe specific treatment—that is discussed in detail under each topic in Section II.

- **Do I need to save a life?**

Answering "yes" means that you must do something *right now* or someone will die. The most common reasons for a "yes" answer are:
1. No heartbeat and/or no breathing
2. Bleeding.

The first must take precedence over the second. First, it takes longer to bleed to death than to die from lack of oxygen to the brain. One to three minutes without oxygen and there is probably serious permanent brain damage; by six minutes you are probably dead. Second, as long as the heart is not beating there is less pressure pumping blood out of a wound. Bleeding will be slower, allowing more time to control it after the heart starts again. Usually all these life-threatening situations won't occur together but, if they do

FIRST start cardiopulmonary resusciation (CPR).

SECOND deal with hemorrhage after breathing and
heartbeat have been restored.

Now, let's assume that the answer to the question was
"yes" and you've solved the problem or that the answer
was "no." In either case it's time for the next question.

- **Do I need to prevent the present situation from getting
worse?**

Has something happened which is no immediate
threat but which could get worse and lead to trouble if I
don't do something to prevent it? Important among the
many possible causes for a "yes" to this question are:
1. Fractures
2. Burns
3. Open wounds
4. Infection
5. Head injury
6. Unconsciousness
7. Exposure to heat or cold
8. Poisoning by mouth or by sting
9. Chest pain.

Again, after you have answered the question "yes" and
taken appropriate action or decided that the answer was
"no" go on to the next question.

- **Do I need to relieve pain and suffering?**

Why pain *and* suffering? Because there are many
forms of suffering other than pain, not the least of which
is fear. A sick or injured person usually feels vulnerable,
anxious, and depressed under any circumstances; at sea,
on a rocking wet boat, a long way from professional help,
these feelings are likely to be many times stronger. After
you have done the procedures or given the drugs recommended for the relief of pain remember that the physical
ailment is happening to a total human being, who may
now need some tender loving care. None of us is so tough
that we are above needing such attention at times. None

of us should feel so hardened as to be unable to give this kind of support. A soft voice, gentle reassurance (even when you are not so "sure" yourself), a hand to hold, a shoulder to cry on can go a long way toward putting a person's mind at ease. Beyond the purely psychological benefits, there is no doubt that a sick body heals better when the mind is at peace.

When necessary, a mild sedative, such as 5 mg. of Valium is helpful. *Never* give it to someone who has been drinking or along with strong painkillers. The combination could be deadly.

At this point, with a combination of planning, a quick review of the guide, some attention to your patient's comfort, and a bit of luck, you are ready for the next question.

- **Do I need help?**

Have I done everything that needs to be done? Will time now bring about a cure or is definitive medical care necessary? At both extremes the answer will be obvious. Most often the medical problems you will face will be minor. Judicious first aid will be all the treatment required. At the other end of the scale, when the answer to the first question has been "yes," it is clear that further medical care, even after the life has been saved, is required. Now the question becomes not "Do I need help?" but "How and where can I get help in a hurry?" The answer will depend on where you are and what means of communication are available to you. It may vary from a fast run to the nearest harbor and a waiting ambulance summoned by radiotelephone to a sea/air rescue by a local Harbor Patrol or Coast Guard unit to a "Mayday" broadcast from midocean accompanied by a prayer that someone with the necessary facilities will hear you and can find you. Between the two extremes lie matters of judgment. How severe is the injury? How serious the illness? How urgent the need for help? How tolerable the pain? In matters of judgment we are all fallible. Often what is credited to superior judgment is no more than the result of more experience with the issue at hand. In such cases do the best that you can with the information and experience that you have.

Section II
Specific Problems
and Suggested
Solutions

Abdominal Pain

A "stomachache" can be a mild discomfort or an excruciating agony. It may result from a trapped gas bubble or from a life-threatening catastrophe. Common causes may include indigestion, food poisoning, a virus infection (stomach "flu"), constipation, appendicitis, kidney stones, gallstones, menstrual cramps, or an ovarian cyst. Until the nature of the problem becomes clear a few simple steps should be followed:

1. Put the patient at rest
2. Do not give food or liquids
3. Do not give laxatives or enemas
4. Give pain medication as needed.

For heartburn or simple indigestion Pepto-Bismol frequently will give quick relief. Follow label directions for dose.

Figuring out the cause of abdominal pain is often very difficult, even for a trained medical professional. Your major concern should be to decide whether the condition is minor and can be dealt with by simple first aid or is potentially dangerous and requires more involved medical or surgical care. The following table gives a few guidelines which may help you to make that judgment. Please remember that these are guidelines only, not absolutes.

Evaluation of Abdominal Pain

Probably Not Serious—First Aid	Possibly Serious—Medical Care
1. Short-lived—less than one day	1. Persistent—more than one day
2. Vomiting occasional	2. Vomiting frequent, persistent
3. Mild to moderate diarrhea (less than 10 stools per day) for less than 2 days	3. Severe diarrhea (more than 10 stools per day), longer than 2 days or bloody stools

4. Generalized, crampy, inter-   4. Localized, sharp
   mittent
5. Soft abdomen, not tender   5. Firm abdomen, tender

In more serious situations, if medical care is more than a day away some additional measures may be necessary.

1. Short-term withholding of food and liquids is fine but over longer periods of time nutrition and, more importantly, hydration must be maintained. Water, juices, tea, or broth are all good. Solid foods should be kept as soft and bland as possible. In general, the more liquids and the fewer solids the better.
2. Very severe pain accompanied by a very hard, tender abdomen may indicate a rupture of an appendix, an ulcer, or an ovarian cyst with the possibility of serious infection. In such cases give 500 mg. Tetracycline every six hours, and continue until professional help is available.

Alcohol in First Aid (uses and abuses)

This is not a lecture on the evils of drink. It is not even an attack on the noble St. Bernard, that legendary purveyor of presumed lifesaving brandy. It is, however, a warning. There is a commonly accepted myth that drinking booze is a good way to keep warm in a very cold environment. Sorry, folks, but it just isn't so! Granted, you *feel* warmer for a while after a nip or two, but that's because alcohol dilates your blood vessels. The extra blood flowing through the many small blood vessels in the skin gives a sensation of surface warmth. At the same time that blood is being chilled by the atmosphere. It then recirculates to your insides, where the chilling of the internal organs, especially the brain, increases the rate of freezing.

Once you are back in a warm environment a drink or two can help to warm you by the reverse process. Of course, some hot tea, coffee, or even a little chicken soup will also do very nicely.

Is there ever a time when the use of whiskey is good first aid. Sure there is! For instance, the high alcohol content can be a great antiseptic if nothing else is available. Pour some on the wound. It smarts, but it works.

A small amount (1 ounce) can be a pretty good sedative and mild painkiller, but *be careful!* Don't give it to anyone who is having trouble breathing and *never* along with other sedatives or tranquilizers. The combination can suppress breathing and kill.

Allergies

A few unlucky people are sensitive to everything. Others seem to tolerate any environment. Still, somewhere, there is probably something which, when eaten, touched or breathed, will trigger an allergic reaction in someone. Stinging insects, such as bees, wasps, and certain species of ants can cause a bad reaction or even death in a susceptible individual. Allergies can affect any part of the body and range from a mild annoyance to a threat to life. Persons with a history of allergy should be prepared with the proper medicine for their usual reactions. Following is an outline of allergic reactions and corresponding suggested treatment.

1. Life-threatening Allergic Reactions
   a. Types
      1) Asthma—severe breathing difficulty with wheezing.
      2) Choking—due to swelling of the tongue or vocal cords.

3) Shock (allergic shock; anaphylactic shock) —all the symptoms of shock: pallor, rapid but weak pulse, shallow respirations, restlessness, anxiety, nausea, vomiting, and, sometimes, sudden death.

b. Treatment
   1) Adrenalin (epinephrine 1/1000) injection, ½ ml.
   2) Decadron injection, 8 mg. (2 ml.).
   3) Lay patient down with head lowered.
   4) Keep warm.
   5) Be prepared to give cardiopulmonary resuscitation (CPR).

2. Non-Life-threatening Allergic Reactions
a. General treatment An antihistamine such as Chlor-Trimeton, 4 mg. every four hours will frequently relieve the discomfort of any allergy.
b. Local treatment
   1) Skin
      a) Eczema—scaling, itching, sometimes weeping. Cool compresses with a solution of 1 tablespoon of baking soda to 8 ounces of water. If very severe, apply a Hydrocortisone lotion or cream after the compress. Repeat every few hours.
      b) Hives—red, itching, irregular, dry swellings. These are inside the skin and local applications usually don't help.
   2) Eyes
      Red, itching, watery, with no pus. Cool compresses and a soothing eye drop like Visine every few hours.
   3) Ears, nose, throat
      Nose drops may make breathing a little easier but should be use sparingly since

they can irritate the nose after a while and
make the symptoms worse.
4) Digestive system
Vomiting, cramps, gas, diarrhea. Treat as
described in entries for Abdominal Pain,
Vomiting, and Diarrhea.

Antibiotics

When the first antibiotic appeared on the scene a
short-lived, half-serious, half-joking one-liner devel-
oped among doctors: "If your patient is sick give penicillin for a day or two. If things don't improve take a history and do a physical." Not very funny and, as things
turned out, not very wise. Despite their great contribu-
tion to the saving of lives, antibiotics have several draw-
backs as well. Many bacteria learn to live with them
and become immune. Some people develop mild to severe allergies to antibiotics. Several antibiotics have potentially serious toxic side effects. Self-treatment with
antibiotics is generally best avoided, but under the conditions of a long ocean passage it may, on occasion, be
necessary. Specific recommendations for the use of antibiotics are discussed in the entries dealing with the
cases to which they apply. Here we present a few general guiding principles.

1. Antibiotics are of *no use at all* against virus or fungus infections. They should be used only in cases
   of proven or strongly suspected bacterial infections, which are potentially dangerous to the patient and which are unlikely to get better if left
   alone.
2. Choice of antibiotic
   In the absence of a laboratory that can identify
   bacteria and determine to which antibiotic they

are sensitive, choosing the correct medication is an educated guessing game. What bacteria are most apt to cause a given disease? Which antibiotics are most likely to kill that germ? If there is more than one choice, which drug has the least possibility of producing harmful side effects?

3. Dose of antibiotics

Doses vary from medication to medication and with the age and weight of the individual. Label directions should be followed carefully. For converting to children's doses see the entry for Children.

4. Duration of treatment

Once the commitment to start an antibiotic is made the medication should be given long enough to eliminate all the infection. Seven to ten days is a minimum for most infections even if the symptoms are gone.

5. Cautions in using antibiotics

a. Always ask about allergies before giving any medicine.

b. Avoid sunlight. Several antibiotics, especially Tetracycline can cause sun sensitivity.

c. Never give Tetracycline to pregnant women or to children under eight years of age. It may cause permanent mottling of the teeth in the child.

d. Rashes, diarrhea, swelling, or vomiting may be allergic reactions and are indications for stopping an antibiotic in most cases.

e. Someone with a serious infection who is apparently not responding to an antibiotic or who is showing signs of allergic reaction to the medication should be considered as an emergency, and appropriate medical care should be sought as soon as possible.

Bleeding
(There is only one pressure point.)

1. Bleeding wounds

   Do you remember all those pressure points in the Scout manuals? Neither do I. No matter, they don't work anyway. There really is only one effective pressure point, and that is directly over the bleeding area. Use something soft, absorbent, and compressible, like cloth or cotton. Sterile material is best. If none is available use the cleanest you can find. On small wounds maintain the pressure until the bleeding stops, then apply a bandage. For larger cuts, which may need stitching or other medical attention, put the pressure on, tie it in place, and leave it until you get to the doctor or decide what further action you will be taking if a doctor is not available (see entry for Cuts). Unless there is massive hemorrhaging it's a good idea to cleanse the wound first, preferably with soap and water.

2. Nosebleeds

   Forget the cold knife to the back of the neck or against the upper gum; they don't work any better than any of the other so-called pressure points. Most nosebleeds will stop if you soak a cloth in cold water, wrap it around the nose, and squeeze the nose tight between the thumb and forefinger. Hold for ten minutes, while the victim breathes through the mouth. As the cloth gets warm, don't remove it; just pour a little more cold water over it. A nosebleed that won't stop with this treatment probably needs packing. With a tweezers push cotton or cloth strips up the nose as far as possible and keep packing until it is tight. If medical care is available, leave the packing in until you get help. If there is no professional help nearby, leave the pack in place at least twenty-four hours, then remove it slowly, being prepared to repeat the procedure if bleeding starts again.

3. Tourniquets

These are dangerous. They cut off circulation to the entire limb, which could conceivably lead to gangrene. Use a tourniquet only when the bleeding is profuse and won't stop with pressure. The choice you make when you apply a tourniquet is between the possible loss of a limb and the certain loss of a life.

To apply a tourniquet wrap a rope, a belt, or a roll of cloth around the limb as close to the wound as possible on the side closest to the heart. Tighten the tourniquet by pulling or twisting as much as necessary to stop the bleeding. Loosen the tourniquet every fifteen to twenty minutes to allow some blood to circulate, then tighten it again. Consider your problem to be an emergency and get help as soon as possible.

Burns
(Take a cold bath.)

Burns are the most painful and potentially most serious of all injuries. There are three degrees of burns:

First Degree
The skin gets red.

Second Degree
The superficial layers of the skin separate, causing blistering and peeling.

Third Degree
The entire thickness of the skin is destroyed, exposing fat and muscle and causing bleeding.

The initial first aid treatment for all degrees of burns is the same: cold water.

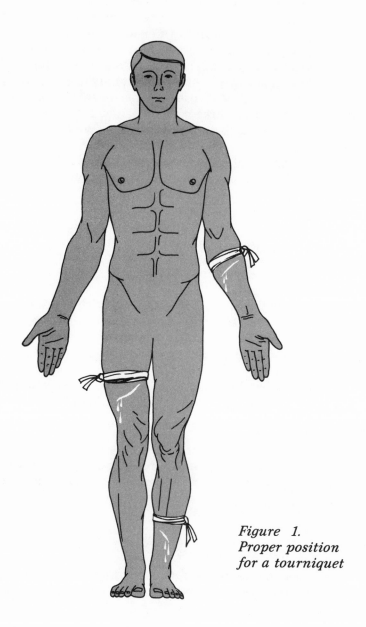

Figure 1.
Proper position
for a tourniquet

If the burned area can be submerged in water, do so. If it cannot be submerged, wrap the area in cloths soaked in cold water. Keep adding water to keep the area cold and wet. Fresh water and sea water are equally good. Don't hold the burn under running water. The force of the water will not only cause pain but may further injure the burned tissue. Don't use creams, ointments, sprays, butter, etc., to any degree of burn. They, too, may cause injury to damaged tissues and create a problem if they need to be removed later.

Follow-up care of burns varies with the degree of the burn and the area of the body surface involved.

1. First degree

   Leave the water on until the pain is gone. If pain returns when the cold application is removed, repeat until the pain is gone for good. First-degree burns rarely require any further treatment.

2. Second degree

   Follow the same procedure as with first-degree burns until the pain has subsided, then apply a layer of sterile Vaseline gauze and cover with a sterile dry dressing. Leave the dressing in place for several days. Do not open blisters; they serve as a protective covering which lessens fluid loss and the danger of infection. Most second-degree burns will heal.

3. Third degree

   All third-degree burns, regardless of size, require follow-up medical and surgical care. Skin grafting is frequently necessary. Until such care is available, follow the same procedure as for second-degree burns.

Life-threatening Burns

1. These are second- or third-degree burns greater than 15 percent of the body (for children or for

adults over sixty make it 10 percent). The palm of an individual's hand is approximately 1 percent of that person's body. The danger is fluid loss through the open skin with the risk of shock. A second hazard is infection. Keep the dressings in place, give as much oral liquids as possible, use medications to relieve pain, and get help *fast!* If more than twenty-four hours will pass before getting help start an antibiotic. Erythromycin (400 mg. every six hours) or Tetracycline (250 mg. every six hours) are good choices.

2. Inhalation of smoke or flame can cause swelling of vocal cords with obstruction to breathing or fluid accumulation in the bronchial tree. The most important first-aid measures are to get the victim away from the smoky area into the fresh air and to give oxygen if it is available. If breathing difficulty does develop give Decadron injection (4 mg.) every four hours.

3. Burns around the genital area can produce swelling, which brings about urinary obstruction. This can be a painful and a serious problem and is not amenable to much in the way of first aid except cold baths.

All three of these situations can rapidly progress beyond the limits of your ability to handle them and should be treated as emergencies as soon as they are recognized, even before obvious serious symptoms develop.

Cardiopulmonary Resuscitation (the ABC's of CPR)

Somewhere, sometime when you least expect it, someone may collapse with cardiac or respiratory arrest. It may result from a heart attack, an electric shock, drowning, or any number of other events. For purposes of first aid it won't matter to you what the cause was; your immediate problem will be the fact that the heart and breathing have stopped.

The treatment of cardiac and respiratory arrest is the same regardless of the cause.

How will you know that there is no heartbeat or that the individual is not breathing? If you know how to feel for a pulse in the neck or can tell if the chest is moving, fine. Don't waste too much time, however. If you see someone limp, blue, and apparently unconscious, assume that an arrest has occurred and start cardiopulmonary resuscitation (CPR). Suppose that you guess wrong and that it wasn't really necessary? You can't do any harm. If you wait too long, however, and it *was* necessary, the price of delay in terms of brain damage is very high. Remember, that first three minutes is critical!

CPR is a skill. It needs to be learned and it needs to be practiced. Good courses are available in most communities. They are usually given by the American Heart Association or by the American Red Cross. Once you know the technique, it's as simple as ABC.

The Technique

1. *Airway*

   When the head tips forward, the tongue falls back into the throat so that air cannot be moved in and out no matter how well you pump. So lay the person on the back. Support the neck with one hand. With the other hand tilt the head back and pull the chin forward. This opens the airway. Wipe any mucus or saliva from the throat with your finger or a cloth. To remove a solid foreign object from the throat use the Heimlich maneuver (see entry for Choking).

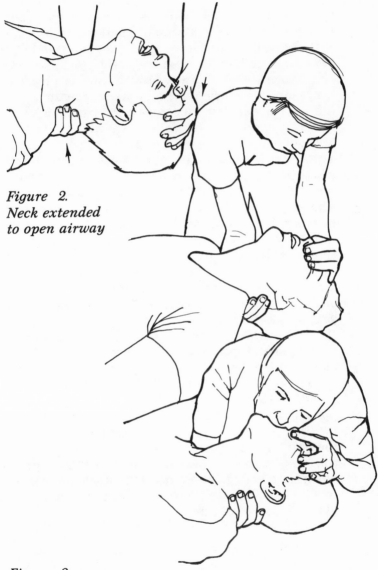

Figure 2.
Neck extended
to open airway

Figure 3.
Proper position for breathing

2. *Breathing*

Supporting the neck with one hand and put your mouth over the victim's mouth, making an airtight seal. Pinch the nose closed with the other hand and blow hard enough to raise the chest one to two inches. Turn your face away toward the chest (so you can watch its movement) and take a breath while the patient exhales, then repeat. Instructions as to how fast and how often follows shortly.

3. *Circulation*

The heart is a little larger than a tennis ball and about as compressible. It lies just behind the sternum (breastplate) and in front of the spinal column. The idea is to squeeze the heart between these two bony structures in order to force the blood out, then to release it, allowing it to rebound to its original shape, which permits blood to flow into the heart again.

Place the victim on a hard surface, such as a table or the floor. A soft surface gives, the spine bends, and you don't get the compression that you need.

Find the lower half of the sternum. The upper end is at the notch between the collarbones. The lower end is where the abdominal muscles start. Find the lower tip of the sternum, measure two fingertip breadths above the tip to avoid breaking it, then place the heel of one hand across the sternum with the fingers raised. The other hand is placed on top of the first hand at right angles to it. lean over the victim and, with your elbows almost straight, press down hard enough to depress the breastplate one to two inches. Quickly release, leaving your hands in place, pause, then repeat.

Rate and Rhythm

Since most people will have adequate circulation at a heart rate between 50 and 100 beats per minute, aim for about 60 compressions per minute. One per second is an

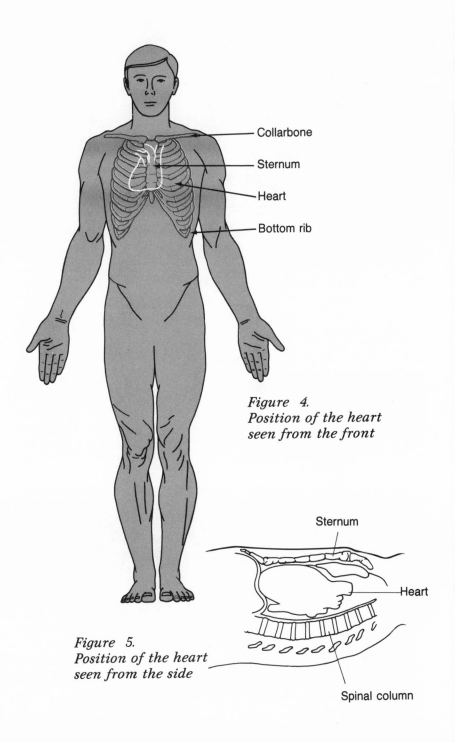

Collarbone

Sternum

Heart

Bottom rib

Figure 4.
Position of the heart
seen from the front

Sternum

Heart

Spinal column

Figure 5.
Position of the heart
seen from the side

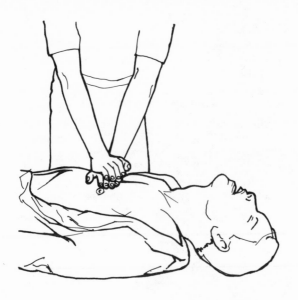

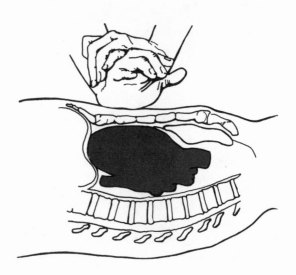

Figure   6.
Proper position for circulation

easy rate to count. Infants under one year of age will require 80 to 100 per minute. For infants use two fingers to compress; for older children use one hand.

With one rescuer, give two breaths one to two seconds apart after each fifteen compressions. With two rescuers, one should do the compression while the other intersperses a breath on the upswing after each fifth compression.

Two rescuers can delay fatigue by periodically quickly shifting positions and exchanging tasks. *Never* interrupt CPR for longer than five seconds.

When to Stop CPR

There are a number of reasons for stopping CPR. Some are easier to accept than others, but all are valid indications for discontinuing.

1. Mission accomplished.
   The victim is responding, breathing spontaneously, the color is improved, and there is a pulse.
2. You've been relieved.
   Someone better equipped, such as a paramedic with resuscitation equipment, is taking over the task.
3. You are physically unable to continue.
   CPR is hard work and we all have limits to our physical endurance.
4. Something else is more important.
   This is the hardest decision to make, but, realistically, certain boat problems could threaten your life and that of other crew members before a victim can be saved.
5. The person is dead.
   Since persons in cardiac and respiratory arrest can often be saved and kept alive for long periods of time, it isn't always easy to know when someone has died. In hospitals sophisticated equipment to

measure brain waves is often used to make the determination. At sea you can only use your judgment. There are two guidelines to follow:

a. If you have reason to believe that the arrest may have occurred more than three or four minutes before you began your efforts and there is no response within a few minutes, there has probably been extensive brain damage and the chances of survival are nil.

b. If you have been able to continue several hours of CPR and there has been no response, the person is almost surely dead. There is only one report of a person surviving after six hours of CPR and only rare cases after three hours.

Summary of CPR

1. Determine consciousness: call to the person and shake him.
2. Open the airway: lift the neck, tilt back the head.
3. Check breathing: place your cheek by the mouth and check the chest for motion.
4. Give four quick breaths: if chest doesn't move, suspect a foreign body. Do the Heimlich maneuver.
5. Feel for pulse in neck: if felt but no breathing, start breathing at one breath per five seconds.
6. If no pulse felt, start CPR: a. One rescuer: two breaths to fifteen compressions
   b. Two rescuers: one breath every fifth compression.

Children
(special problems and
considerations)

In some ways children are just small adults; in many other ways they are a breed apart. For the cruising family a few guides to the emergency medical care of youngsters is in order.

1. Emergency first aid

    Most of the time the same procedures recommended for adults will be appropriate for children.

2. Fever

    Children frequently develop much higher fevers than adults in response to minor illnesses. The kind and intensity of other symptoms are better indicators of the severity of a child's illness than the level of the temperature.

3. Dehydration

    The smaller the child, the less the tolerance for fluid loss through vomiting, diarrhea, or excessive perspiration. Adequate fluid replacement early is important. One and one-half to 2 ounces of liquid per pound of body weight per twenty-four hours is a good average. If fluid loss seems to be greater and signs of dehydration are developing (dry mouth, circles under the eyes, pale skin, listlessness, and decreased urinating), the amount can be increased. A mixture of 10 teaspoons of sea water to one quart of fresh water can be used.

4. Poisoning

    See entry for poisoning.

5. Medications

    Most medicines used for children are available in liquid form. Unfortunately, many of them have a very limited shelf life in that form. Before families cruise long distances, it is a good idea to check with a doctor for advice on which medicines to carry in what form.

    Have a written list of doses for the size (in weight) and age of each child aboard. In a situation in which only adult dosage forms and information are available, you can be reasonably safe in using a dose-to-weight ratio. Here is how it works:

Drug dosage for children.

a. Consider the average adult to weigh 150 pounds.
b. A 15-pound child would then be given 1/10 of the adult dose, a 30-pound child 1/5, a 50-pounder 1/3, and so on.
c. If the weight of the child is such that the calculated dose exceeds the recommended adult dose, do not give more than the adult dose. There are some very fat children, especially among preteens, and the situation will sometimes arise.
d. The task of dividing a capsule or a tablet designed for adult use into a size appropriate for a child may seem formidable. Try this trick: Crush the tablet to a powder or empty the contents of a capsule. Completely dissolve the entire amount into a carefully measured small volume of water. Now the proper fraction of the liquid should contain the desired amount of the medication. For example:
    1) Adult dose = 500 mg. Drug is available in 500 mg. tablet or capsule.
    2) Child weighs 50 pounds. The desired dose is thus 1/3 of the adult dose, or 166 mg.
    3) Dissolve 500 mg. into 3 teaspoons.
    4) One teaspoon now contains the right dose.

Choking
(the Heimlich maneuver)

Hundreds of people die every year from choking on a solid object caught in the throat. The most common cause is a piece of meat. A recent study showed that most of the victims also had high blood alcohol levels and were in a social setting, such as a party or restaurant. It would appear that drinking too much, talking too much, and eating too fast can be a deadly combination.

How will you know that someone is choking? There are several giveaway clues.

1. Hand clutching the throat.
2. Can't talk, can't breathe, can't cough.
3. Skin color getting pale or blue.

Quick action is imperative. The most effective method for dislodging a foreign object from the throat is to use

2071867

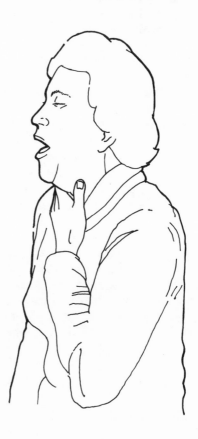

Figure 7.
Typical appearance
of a choking victim

the maneuver first described by Dr. Henry Heimlich. Remember the old popguns that kids used to play with? You pushed hard on the plunger at one end of a tube and a cork in the other end popped out. Well, that's the idea. You push hard on the abdomen and the pressure forces the foreign body out of the throat. There are two steps to the Heimlich maneuver.

1. Back thumps to dislodge the object.
2. Abdominal thrusts to force it out.
   Deliver back thumps with the closed fist between the shoulder blades.
   Abdominal thrusts are given in the midline between the lower end of the sternum (breastplate) and the navel.
The procedure, depending on the victim, goes like this:

1. Conscious adult
   a. 4 back thumps
   b. 4 abdominal thrusts. Stand behind the person, wrap your arms around the middle in a bear hug, place the thumb side of one fist against the abdomen, place the other hand over the fist, and pull firmly in and up.
   c. Repeat the sequence until the object is out.

2. Unconscious adult
   a. Roll the person on the side, facing you, and give 4 back thumps.
   b. Roll him or her onto the back and with your crossed open hands press in hard and repeatedly on the abdomen.
   c. Repeat this sequence until the choking is relieved.

3. Child over one year of age
   a. Place the child over your lap, head down, give 4 back thumps.

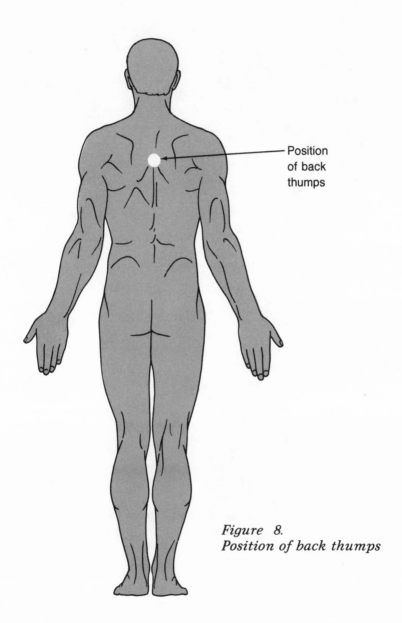

Position
of back
thumps

Figure 8.
Position of back thumps

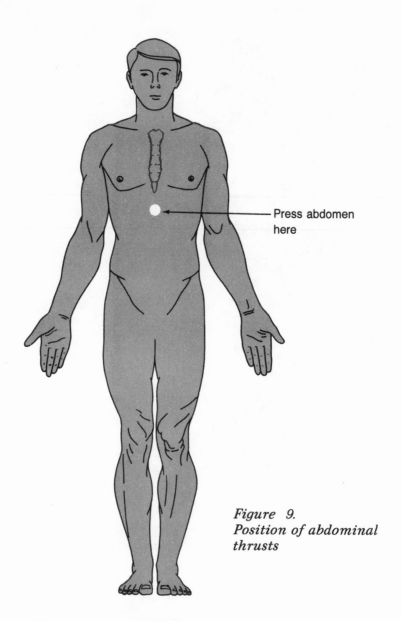

Press abdomen
here

Figure 9.
Position of abdominal
thrusts

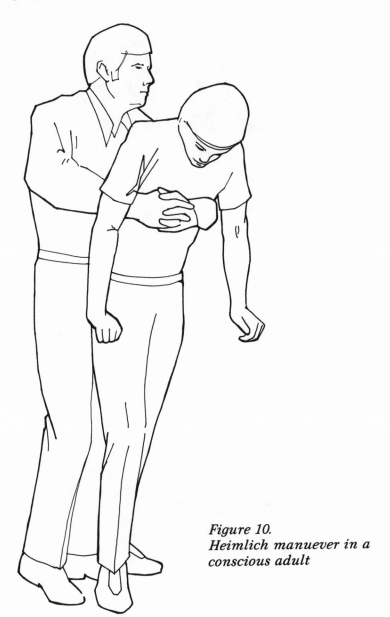

Figure 10.
Heimlich manuever in a
conscious adult

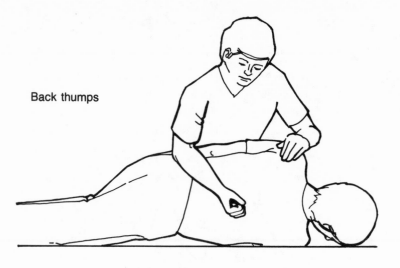

Back thumps

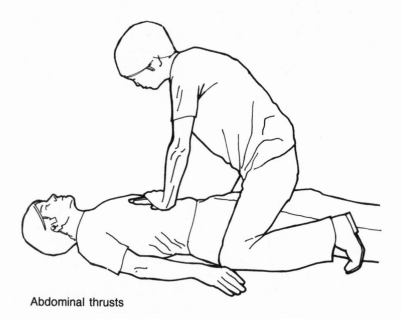

Abdominal thrusts

Figure 11.
Heimlich manuever in an unconscious adult

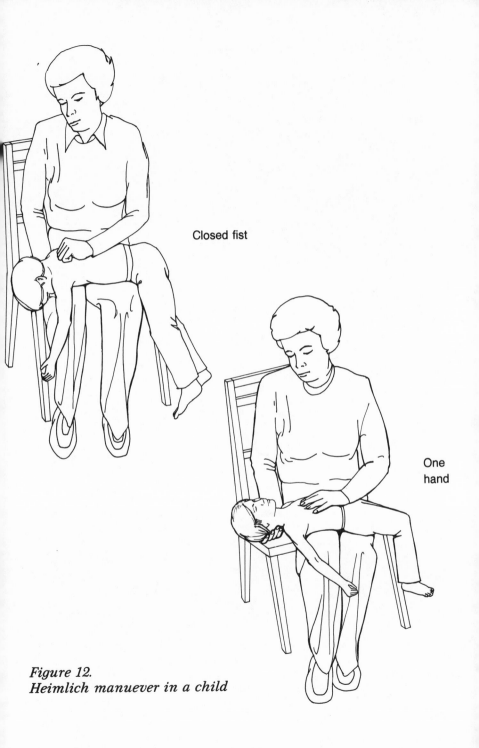

Closed fist

One hand

Figure 12.
Heimlich manuever in a child

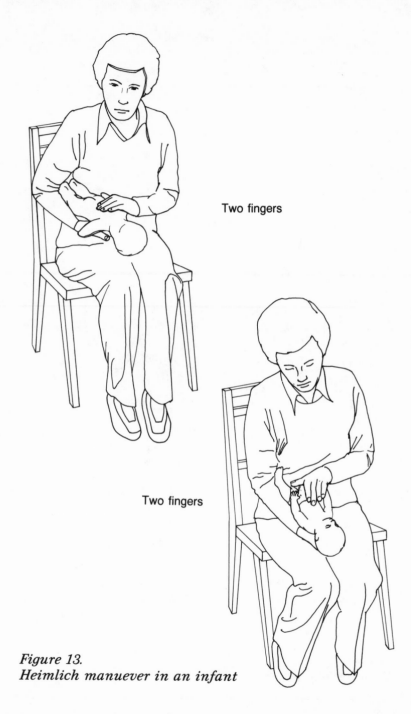

Two fingers

Two fingers

Figure 13.
Heimlich manuever in an infant

  b. Roll the youngster onto the back, still on your
     lap, and give 4 abdominal thrusts with one
     hand.
  c. Repeat the sequence as often as necessary.

4. Infant under one year of age.
   a. Hold the baby face down on your arm and give
      4 back thumps with 2 fingers.
   b. Roll the baby over face up on your arm and give
      4 abdominal thrusts with 2 fingers.
   c. Repeat the sequence until successful.

Cold

The effects of exposure to cold can range from a little
local frostnip to death by freezing. They are all easier to
prevent than to correct:

1. Wear warm clothes that are not too tight.
2. Keep hands, feet, and head covered; a lot of heat can
   be lost through the exposed surfaces even if the rest
   of of you is well covered.
3. Get out of wet clothes as soon as possible.
4. Drink warm liquids and eat warm food; they help to
   warm the blood as it circulates through the gut.
5. Avoid cold drinks and *stay away from booze!* (see
   entry for Alcohol in First Aid).

Cold Injuries and Their Treatment

1. Frostnip
   Wind and below-freezing temperatures cause
   numb white patches on exposed skin, especially
   on the face. A face mask, a good face cream, or
   sunscreen cream can help to protect against this.
   If frostnip does appear, get into a warm place as

soon as possible. Until you can get in out of the cold, blowing on the area or sheltering it in a warm place inside the clothing is helpful. Do not wash or rub the area. A few blisters and a couple of days of numbness are probably the worst you can expect.

2. Frostbite

As cold progresses and persists, unless something is done, blood vessels, nerves, and muscles start to be damaged. Constricting blood vessels cut down circulation, especially to nose, ears, and the ends of fingers and toes. Redness and burning go on to numbness and whitening of the skin over large areas.

The best treatment is rapid rewarming in warm water baths at temperatures of 104° to 108° F. (40° to 42° C). This temperature range will feel barely lukewarm to a normal hand. As the tissues thaw they will hurt terribly and you may need to use your strongest pain medication or sedative (see entry for Pain). As the thawing progresses, blistering may develop. Leave the blisters alone. Keep the injured part at rest. Put sterile cotton pads between the fingers or toes. Follow-up medical care is usually necessary because of tissue damage. Until help is available a warm soak twice a day for about twenty minutes may prevent further damage or infection.

3. Freezing

When the body is exposed to cold, the blood circulating through the skin gets chilled. As it passes to the internal body structures it cools them. If the exposure continues, the body temperature drops and the function of vital organs, especially the brain, is depressed. The freezing person tends to gradually get drowsy, lose judgment, fall asleep, slip into coma, and die.

The greatest freezing hazard to the sailor is going

overboard in a cold sea. Survival time in cold water is surprisingly short; statistics show an average of seven hours at 60° F. to one and one-half hours at 32° F. Recent research studies done at the University of Victoria, British Columbia, have demonstrated a few ways of prolonging significantly that survival time. The Canadian researchers have reported as long as 50 percent increase in survival time by the use of these two simple measures:

   a. Dress warmly when sailing in cold waters. Particularly have hands, feet, head, armpits, and groin well covered with extra warm layers; those are the areas of maximum heat loss.

   b. If you are in the water, unless you are just minutes of swimming time from safety, don't try to swim or move around a lot. Curl up in a fetal position and float quietly. Here's where a good float coat or life jacket is important. The more you move about the more blood circulates to your arms and legs, gets chilled by the surrounding water, and circulates back inside, and the sooner you will freeze to death.

Freezing, to any degree, is treated the same way; get the body warm, inside and out, as quickly as possible.

   a. Get wet clothes off.

   b. Wrap in warm blankets.

   c. Give warm liquids to drink.

   d. If the person is unconscious, don't try to pour liquids into the the mouth; it can cause choking. Warm water can be given rectally with an enema syringe.

   e. If the total environment is very cold, bundling together in a blanket or sleeping bag with a person of normal temperature can help to warm the frozen body fairly quickly.

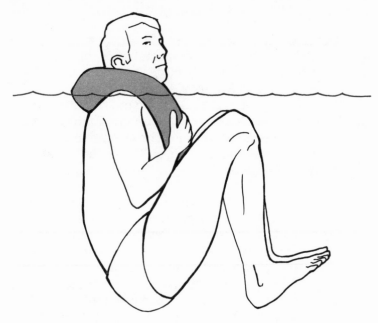

Figure 14.
Floating fetal position

Compresses
(hot packs or cold packs—when to use which)

Understanding the effects of hot and cold when applied locally will eliminate the confusion that frequently arises over the indications for using one or the other.

Cold causes small blood vessels to constrict, thereby decreasing the flow of blood to the area. It also numbs nerve endings, producing a local anesthetic effect.

Heat dilates the small blood vessels so that the flow of blood is increased.

Immediately after an injury we are interested in easing pain and in minimizing bleeding and swelling. The application of cold serves these functions.

After one or two hours, when the acute pain has subsided, the bleeding is controlled, and the maximum swelling has occurred, we want to speed the reduction of swelling and to promote the healing of injured tissue. The fluid which produces swelling is removed by reabsorption into the blood stream. In addition, much of the healing process is carried on by components of the blood. Increasing blood flow enhances these activities, so local heat is indicated.

Thus the simple rule following an injury is:

EARLY . . . . . cold

LATE . . . . . . heat

Since the blood also has many bacteria-fighting elements, increasing blood flow to an infection can speed healing. Warm compresses are, therefore, good for local infection.

Constipation

Modern society seems to worship at the shrine of the regular bowel movement. Fortunes are spent in the marketing and consumption of laxatives. This preoccupation is, for the most part, based on folklore. True constipation, however, which is a frequent unwelcome visitor aboard a sailing vessel, can be very distressing. Constipation should be defined as a condition in which the stools are sufficiently hard or infrequent to be the cause of abdominal discomfort or of painful, difficult bowel movements. A few simple measures will usually prevent the problem from developing.

1. Drink adequate liquids.
2. Eat fruit and vegetables when they are available.

3. Don't overdo some of the common "binding" foods, such as cheese, chocolate, nuts, bananas, apples, and tea.
4. Don't ignore the urge to have a bowel movement just because going to the head is inconvenient or uncomfortable. The longer feces stay in the bowel the more water is absorbed from them and the harder they are to pass.
5. Don't hurry your head call. Eliminate as much as possible at each sitting.
6. For the constipation-prone individual, a nonlaxative stool softener taken regularly is helpful. Mineral oil or Haley's M-O work well, but are messy and hard to carry. Colace capsules are usually effective and can safely be used indefinitely. Start with one capsule three times a day and increase or decrease to achieve the desired result.
7. Don't use laxatives. All laxatives act by irritating the intestines; not only do they frequently cause cramps, but they may also produce a reflex relaxation of the intestinal wall that leads to the need for more laxatives later.

If constipation does develop, one of the following will usually give relief:

1. A glycerin suppository inserted into the rectum.
2. A Fleet enema (pediatric strength for children).
3. A warm water enema. Eight to 16 ounces (half as much for children) by bulb syringe or enema bag will work very well.

If none of the above measures are successful medical attention may be required, although constipation rarely develops to that point, if attended to early.

Convulsions
(fits and seizures)

Terrible to experience and frightening to behold, a convulsion is a more or less widely distributed, unnatural, violent, and involuntary spasm or series of spasms of the muscles usually accompanied by a temporary loss of consciousness. The causes include epilepsy and a variety of insults to the brain. Physical trauma, excess heat or cold, infections, poisons, oxygen deprivation, tumors, and, especially in young children, high fever may trigger a seizure. Regardless of the origin of the fit, which needs to be evaluated and dealt with in its own right, the convulsion itself is most often a self-limited event of several seconds' to a few minutes' duration, which requires no treatment. The persistent or recurrent convulsion calls for the use of medications and techniques beyond the limits of the nonprofessional and is an emergency. The disease leading to the convulsion may be very serious or relatively benign, but the seizure itself rarely causes serious aftereffects and almost never kills.

The most important service you can render is to protect the individual from injury during the attack:

1. Put the patient in a position where he or she will not be hurt by falling or striking a flailing arm, leg, or head against a hard surface.
2. Do not restrain the individual. The strength of the muscle spasm is very great; joints have been dislocated and bones broken straining against strong bonds.
3. Prevent choking. The tongue will frequently fall back into the throat. Tilting the head back lifts the tongue up and prevents obstruction to the airway.
4. After the seizure is over, let the person rest or sleep while you systematically evaluate the possible causes and decide your course of action.

Cuts

The treatment of a cut of any size involves several goals:

1. Stop bleeding

   Apply pressure to the wound until the bleeding stops. This subject is discussed in greater detail in the entry for Bleeding.

2. Prevent infection

   Cleanse the cut thoroughly with soap and water or a good antiseptic such as Betadine. When you have finished whatever additional treatment is necessary put on a sterile bandage large enough to cover the cut and at least ½ inch of intact skin around it.

3. Preserve function

   Always check to see that the part of the body which has been cut works properly. For example, does a finger bend and straighten as it should? If it does not, a nerve or tendon may be severed. There isn't anything that you can do about that immediately. Go ahead and treat the wound as you normally would, but every effort should be made to get surgical care as soon as possible.

4. Promote healing and minimize scarring

   Cuts heal from side to side, not from end to end. It is less important how long or deep a laceration is than how wide it is. In order for healing to occur with the least amount of scarring it is necessary to keep the edges as close together as possible. Often just placing the injured part in a relaxed position will let the edges come together. If motion, such as bending a joint, separates the edges, a splint at the joint will frequently do the trick.

Sometimes there is enough tension on a wound that the edges will not lie together. If the pull is not too strong, steristrips or butterfly bandages work very well to hold the cut closed.

   a. Steri-Strips
These are adhesive paper strips packaged in a sterile plastic container which is opened by pulling apart its ends. The steristrips are on a piece of cardboard which is perforated near one end.

To apply Steri-Strips follow these steps:

   1) Open the steristrip package by pulling apart the ends.
   2) Tear off the shorter end of the cardboard backing.
   3) Lift one steristrip at a time by its end.
   4) Press the end against the skin on one side of the cut, pull across the cut to bring the edges together, then press down on the other side of the wound.

   b. Butterfly bandages
These are packaged like Band-Aids. Their shape gives them their name. Open the package in the usual way and apply, using the same procedure as for steristrips.

Wounds in which the gap is too wide or the tension too great to allow the above procedures to work will require stitching. In such cases, cleanse the wound, stop the bleeding, apply a sterile dressing, and get to a doctor as soon as possible. The longer the delay, the greater the risk of infection or bad scarring. The long-distance sailor, many days away from medical care, may want to try suturing at sea. It has been done successfully many times. If you are so inclined, solicit the help of a physician or check with a local emergency hospital now. Learn what equipment is needed, the basics of sterile technique, and the actual sewing procedure. It isn't all that hard, but it cannot be learned by reading. If the idea of sewing up a cut seems a little too much for you, don't fault yourself. You will have reached one of the legitimate limits of your ability.

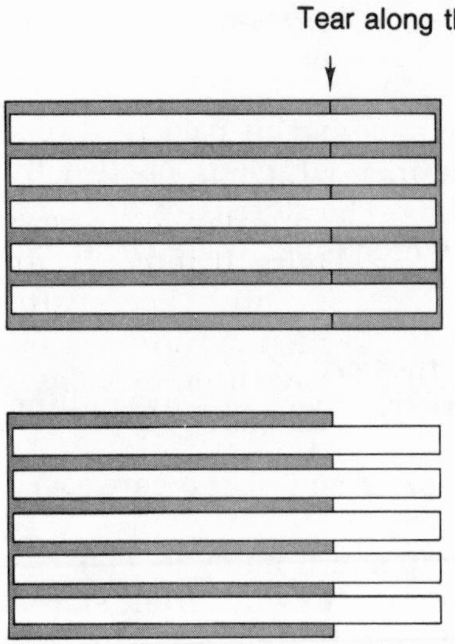

Tear along this line

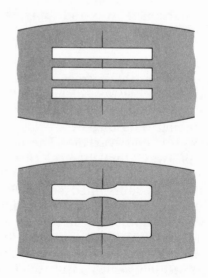

Figure 15.
Steri-Strips

Figure 16.
Steri-strips and butterfly bandages in place

The Infected Cut

If a laceration is very dirty or if signs of infection, such as redness, local heat, swelling, or tenderness appear, and medical attention is more than a day away, start Erythromycin, 400 mg. every six hours. If infection appears to be getting worse or is not getting better after twenty-four to forty-eight hours, switch to Nafcillin, 500 mg. every four hours. When there have been no signs of infection for twenty-four hours or longer, you can stop the drug.

Diarrhea

The discomfort and the inconvenience of frequent watery bowel movements are unpleasant enough at any time. Within the confines of a small boat they can be intolerable. In addition, the loss of water and minerals from the body over a prolonged period of time without adequate replacement can be devastating and sometimes fatal. Diarrhea is a symptom, not a disease. There are many possible causes:

1. Dietary indiscretion
   This is probably the most common cause. You ate too much, you drank too much. The diarrhea is usually mild and short-lived.
2. Virus infections ("stomach flu")
   This is undoubtedly next in line in frequency of causes for diarrhea. There may be low-grade fever, headache, muscle pain, and other "virus" symptoms. The average duration is one to three days.
3. Food "poisoning"
   This is not really poisoning. The term is generally applied to indicate an infection from bacterially contaminated food. The diarrhea may be more severe and accompanied by high fever.

4. Specific dysentery

There is a form of severe, profuse, frequently bloody diarrhea, usually accompanied by high fever, abdominal pain, and creating a very sick, toxic patient, which is the result of infection of the bowel with one of several organisms with exotic names, such as *Salmonella, Entamoeba histolytica, Vibrio cholera, Shigella,* and several others. The source of infection is almost always contaminated food or water. This group of diseases is potentially life-threatening and requires intensive medical care involving intravenous fluids and, in some cases, specific anti-infectious medication.

Careful attention to prevention of these diseases is, therefore, essential. While traveling in places where sanitation is suspect, take a few simple precautions.

1. Boil the water at least twenty minutes.
2. Wash all food thoroughly.
3. Cook all food, including fruits and vegetables.
4. If you must eat something raw, peel it.

Treatment of Diarrhea

1. Fluids

The primary danger with diarrhea is excessive loss of body fluids and minerals. It's important to keep up the oral fluid intake. Water, apple juice, clear soup, nonfat milk diluted with equal parts of water are usually well tolerated and adequate for mild diarrhea. If loose stools are very large, very frequent, or persist for a prolonged period of time, dehydration may develop, and dehydration is a serious illness in its own right. Some of the signs of early dehydration are dry mouth, decreased urination, hot dry skin, circles under the eyes, a "fruity" acetone smell to the breath, and increasing listlessness. The appearance of any of these symptoms is an indication to head for a place where intravenous fluids can be given. At sea, when such a facility is too far away, you can try an alternative method of replacing water and minerals by mouth. Mix 10 teaspoons of sea water with one full quart of fresh water. Give an adult 3 to 4 quarts per twenty-four hours in small frequent amounts. For a child under 65 pounds 1½ to 2 ounces per pound per twenty-four hours is an average amount. If diarrhea is profuse and signs of dehydration are increasing, the amount of fluid can be increased.

2. Nonspecific medications

Except for some of the specific dysenteries, it is doubtful that medication is of any value in curing diarrhea. There are several preparations which may offer relief of some of the discomfort and slow down the frequency of head calls. There is some possibility that using these medications is unwise because the infected material is kept in the intestine longer and prolongs the disease, but it's hard to be a purist when you feel lousy, and most people will opt for some relief.

a. Kaopectate

I, personally, don't believe it is of much use, but some people swear by it. It is inexpensive and harmless and 3–6 tablespoons every three or four hours for adults or one tablespoon for children may soothe a mildly aching gut.

b. Pepto-Bismol

This used to be considered in the same league with Kaopectate until a recent study showed that it may be the very best treatment for the *turistas* so common to the traveler in many Latin American countries. The dose is 1 to 2 ounces every half hour for eight doses.

c. Lomotil

This very popular drug requires a prescription. It slows down intestinal activity, thus reducing cramps and lessening diarrhea temporarily. There are potential undesirable side effects, and dosage instructions must be followed carefully.

For adults: 2 tablets 3 to 4 times a day for 1 to 2 days, then 1 tablet every 12 hours.

For children: use the liquid form. Never give to children under two years.
2 to 5 years: 1 teaspoon every 8 hours.
5 to 8 years: 1 teaspoon every 6 hours.
8 to 12 years: 1 teaspoon every 5 hours.

3. Specific medications

In the presence of high fever with profuse or bloody diarrhea there may be reason to suspect a specific dysentery. Consider ten or more stools a day to be a profuse diarrhea. Unless facilities for making a proper diagnosis are reasonably close at hand, it would be wise to start antibiotic treatment. Give 500 mg. ampicillin every six hours. Ampicillin is a cousin to penicillin, so be sure to ask about penicillin allergy. Do not let the use of this medication be a substitute for follow-up medical care as soon as possible. The long-range complications of some of the specific dysenteries can be quite serious.

Ears

All ear pain is not the same. Different kinds of discomfort come from different causes and each requires its own specific treatment.

1. The ear hurts to touch

Lying on the ear or tugging the outer ear is painful. Water in the ear burns and stings. These symptoms usually indicate an infection of the lining of

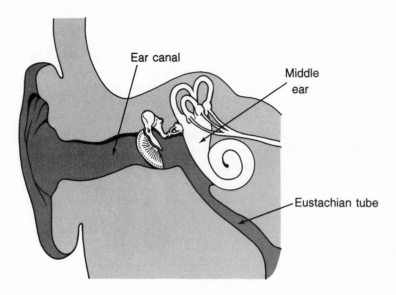

Figure 17.
The anatomy of the ear viewed from the front

the ear canal, the so-called "swimmer's ear." It is commonly a mixed infection with fungus and bacteria, not unlike athlete's foot. The treatment is Cortisporin otic solution. Put five drops in the ear followed by a small piece of cotton moistened with the drops. Repeat, using fresh cotton, four times a day until there is no pain for two to three days. Recurrences can often be prevented by putting rubbing alcohol in each ear and letting it soak for one or two minutes after swimming.

2. The ear feels plugged

There is a sense of fullness and pressure deep in the ear. Hearing is decreased. There is no pain when the ear is moved or pressed. Most likely there has been an increase in pressure in the nose from diving, descent from altitude, or congestion of the nose. Air has been forced up the Eustachian tube and is trapped in the middle ear (see Figure 17). There are several tricks for opening the tube and relieving the pressure.

    a. Yawn.

    b. Drink liquids.

    c. Chew gum.

    d. Use decongestant nose drops or a decongestant nasal spray.

    e. Blow up a balloon or blow into the back of your hand with a little pressure.

    f. Compress your nose between your thumb and forefinger and *gently* blow until you feel your ear "pop."

3. There is sharp persistent pain inside the ear

There are probably also all the discomforts associated with a plugged Eustachian tube, but now there is severe pain as well, not related to moving the outer ear. This probably means infection in the middle ear, a very common ailment in children, relatively infrequent in adults. If there is also fever, sore throat, or a cold, you can be more sure of infection, but an ear infection can exist without these other complaints. Middle ear infections need antibiotic treatment. Use ampicillin. The adult dose is 500 mg. every six hours. For children under forty pounds, give 10 mg. per pound of body weight every six hours. For example, a 25-pound child would get 125 mg. every six hours.

The ampicillin (or penicillin)-allergic patient should take Erythromycin. The adult dose is 400 mg. every six hours. Children take 5 mg. per pound of body weight every six hours.

It is important to continue treatment for ten full days even if all the symptoms are gone to be sure that the infection is completely eliminated. If medical attention is available by the time treatment is complete, it is a good idea to have the ear checked for possible residual infection.

Eyes

So precious and so vulnerable, our eyes deserve some tender loving care and protection from the many hazards that threaten them.

1. Sun
    The rays of the sun, especially when reflected from the water, can cause severe eyestrain and sometimes even damage the inside of the eye, leading to temporary or permanent loss of vision. Good sunglasses are important. Polarized lenses are the best. The tint should be dark enough to cut the glare. Once burned, treatment may do little to correct the damage. Cold compresses and eye patches are all that can be done as first aid. Even in the hands of an eye specialist, the condition may not be reversible.
2. Irritants
    Wind and water can make your eyes very sore and more susceptible to infection. Face masks or goggles will help to prevent irritation. Cold compresses and a mild eye drop, like Visine, will usually give relief.
3. Infections (conjunctivitis, pinkeye)
    The eye becomes red, tears a lot, and frequently has a discharge of pus. Gentle washing with warm water followed by a drop of 10 percent Sulamyd eye solution every four hours will clear most cases. Continue treatment until twenty-four to forty-eight hours after the eyes look and feel normal. If the eye does not clear in a day or two, there may be

a more serious infection, which could threaten vision. Early medical attention is important.

4. Foreign bodies
   a. Loose foreign bodies
      Most small objects which get into the eye float on the surface. Flushing with lots of water will usually wash them out.
   b. Stuck foreign bodies
      Stubborn bits stuck to the inside of the lid can usually be wiped away very gently with a wisp of cotton or the corner of a handkerchief.
      To expose a foreign object under the lower lid pull the lid down while the victim rolls the eyes up.
      The upper lid can be curled back over a Q-tip or a toothpick while the victim rolls the eyes down.
   c. Imbedded foreign bodies
      If the object does not rinse or wipe away readily, it may have penetrated the surface of the eye. Removing these requires special instruments and special skills. Keep the eye covered and get help as soon as possible. If help will not be available within twenty-four hours, put one drop of Sulamyd eye solution in the eye every four hours to prevent infection.

Fever

Fever is a symptom which causes many people a great deal of unnecessary anxiety. A review of fever's causes and effects may help to put it in perspective.

What Is Fever?

Fever is an elevation of body temperature above "normal." Normal is the usual range of body temperature for a given individual when there is no illness. It may vary from person to person, but generally fluctuates within a degree above or below 98.6° F. (37° C.) when taken by mouth, one degree higher in the rectum and one degree lower under the arm. The choice of location for taking the temperature is a matter of personal preference, convenience, or practicality. It is important, however, to be aware of the differences in normal level at each site in order to evaluate any given temperature reading. Generally, oral temperature between 96° F. and 99° F. can be considered normal in adults. Temperatures in children are usually a little higher, so that 100° F. would be the upper limit of normal.

The metric system and metric thermometers are in common use in many places. The following table shows the relationship between Fahrenheit and Celsius temperatures in the usual range found in humans.

Fahrenheit	Celsius
98.6	37.0
100.0	37.8
100.4	38.0
101.0	38.3
102.0	38.9
103.0	39.0
104.0	40.0
105.0	40.6

How Is Fever Measured?

A fever thermometer is calibrated in the range of usual body temperature. It has a locking mechanism which permits mercury to rise to the temperature level being recorded but not to fall again unless shaken vigorously. The tip may be elongated, as in an oral thermometer, or blunt, as in a rectal thermometer.

Theoretically, the long tip is easier to place under the tongue, while the blunt tip is less likely to break

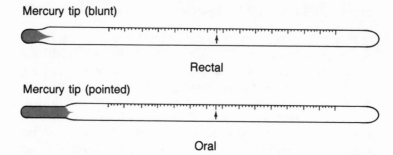

Mercury tip (blunt)

Rectal

Mercury tip (pointed)

Oral

Figure 18.
Rectal and oral thermometers

off in the rectum. The real reason for the difference is
more likely for identification; it helps to avoid the
unaesthetic and unsanitary practice of taking oral
temperatures with a thermometer which was previ-
ously used rectally. The calibrations and reading of
the two are identical.

Using the Thermometer

1. Cleanse the thermometer thoroughly with soap and
   water or alcohol.
2. Hold the thermometer by the end away from the
   mercury tip and shake vigorously until the reading is several degrees below normal.
3. Insert the mercury tip under the tongue, in the rectum, or under the arm. For insertion into the rectum lubricate the tip with a small amount of Vaseline. Leave the thermometer in place for three
   minutes.
4. Holding the thermometer only by the end away
   from the mercury tip, rotate the thermometer
   back and forth until you can see the mercury
   column. Holding the mercury tip can raise the
   reading. Read the temperature at the end of the
   mercury column.

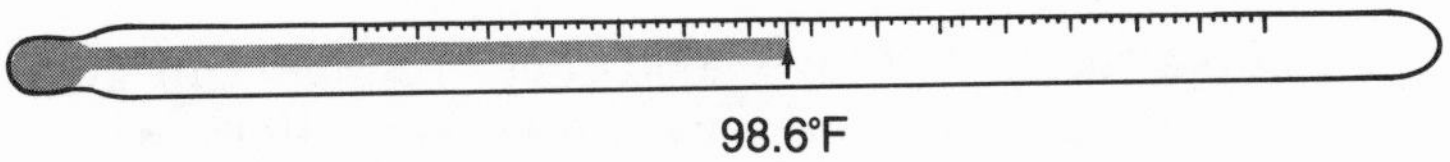

98.6°F

Figure 19. Reading the thermometer

What Does Fever Mean?

Fever is a clue that the body is not well. The most common cause of fever is infection, but dehydration, overexposure to sun or heat, and certain metabolic diseases may also cause the body temperature to go up. The degree of fever does not necessarily indicate the seriousness of the cause; minor or severe illnesses may be accompanied by high or low fevers.

Is Fever Dangerous?

The fever itself is rarely dangerous. The worst effect of fever is usually the discomfort which goes along with it. Prolonged fever causes loss of body fluid through perspiration and through the water vapor in the air we exhale as we breathe rapidly, so it is important to increase fluid intake when the body temperature is high. Fevers of 105° F. or higher are potentially harmful to the brain and the heart. Some effort should be made to reduce fever to a level below 104° F.

How Is Fever Treated?

1. Medication

Aspirin and acetaminophen (Tylenol, Datril, Tempra, Phenaphen) are the most commonly used fever-reducing drugs. There is probably not much difference between them in benefit or in undesired side effects. Both are good fever reducers in normal doses and both are potential killers when overused. Ten grains of either medication every four hours is a good average dose for adults and should not be exceeded. *Increasing the dose does not increase the benefits but does increase the hazards.*

2. Cool sponge baths

   As with any hot object, applying cool water will lower the temperature. The water should be slightly cool. Except for dangerously high levels (see entry for Heat), avoid ice packs or ice-cold tubs. They may result in chills and are too shocking to the system.

3. Dress lightly

   You don't cool hot objects by wrapping them in insulating materials. If a chill accompanies the fever it may be necessary to bundle the patient up warmly until the chill subsides, but as soon as shivering and the cold feeling are gone take the wrappings off.

Fever of Unknown Cause

Whenever possible, identify and treat the underlying cause of the fever. When this is not possible, a judgment must be made as to whether or not to use antibiotics. If fever is low grade (less than 102° F.) and the patient does not appear to be very sick, you can safely just treat symptoms for several days. In a very sick individual, or in the presence of very high fever, with no apparent diagnosis and no medical care available, it is probably wise to start an antibiotic.

Ampicillin (check penicillin allergy first), 500 mg. every six hours, or Erythromycin, 400 mg. every six hours, are good choices. If after forty-eight hours of one medication there is no improvement, try the other. Continue the one which is helping for at least ten days. If neither helps, it's time to think of emergency medical care.

Fractures and Sprains
(When in doubt, immobilize.)

Sometimes fractures are easy to identify. An arm or a leg is bent at an unnatural angle or the broken ends of the bone can be seen or felt. More often, it is very difficult to distinguish between a fracture and a sprain. Swelling, pain, bluish discoloration, and pain with motion may be present with either. Often only an X ray will show the difference. X ray is rarely available at the scene of an accident and at sea may be many days away. For purposes of immediate first aid, it isn't important to tell a fracture from a sprain. Immobilization, ice packs for pain, and the use of pain medication is equally good treatment for both.

Types of Fracture

1. Simple fractures
   Despite the name, a simple fracture may at times be quite complex. The term is used to describe a fracture in which the skin is intact so that there is no communication between the bone and the outside. Simple fractures may be:
   a. Incomplete (greenstick)
      The bone is broken part way through. The unbroken portion holds the bone together and in position. This is the safe and easy kind.
   b. Complete
      The bone is broken into two or more parts. The pull of muscles on the broken pieces causes distortion and there is usually a noticeable deformity. There are two risks with this

type of fracture: disability due to improper position of healing; and injury to nerves or blood vessels by the broken bone ends.

2. Compound fractures

This term refers to a complete fracture in which the skin is broken as well, so that the broken bone is in contact with the outside. The compound fracture carries the additional risk of infection to the bone.

Treatment of Fracture

The immediate first aid treatment for any fracture or sprain is the same.

1. Help the injured person to a comfortable position of rest.

2. Apply ice packs to the affected area.

This helps to reduce swelling and relieve pain. The packs can be left on for several hours if the patient does not need to be moved.

3. Give pain medication (see entry for Pain).

Getting the injured part into a position where it can be immobilized can be a difficult and painful procedure and will require as much relaxation and cooperation from the injured party as possible.

4. Immobilize the injured part.

Don't rush! After the ice and the pain medication have had time to make the victim more comfortable, *slowly* start to move the arm or leg into position for splinting. Remember that you are not trying to set a broken bone into a normal position. You are merely trying to immobilize it. Be careful not to apply too much pressure or you might injure a nerve or blood vessel with the sharp end of the bone in the case of a complete fracture.

If you have appropriate splints for the part of the body which has been injured, use them. Be sure to

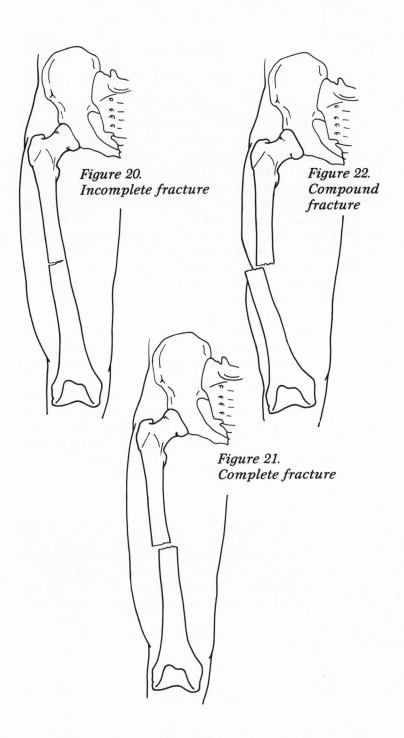

Figure 20.
Incomplete fracture

Figure 22.
Compound
fracture

Figure 21.
Complete fracture

secure the splint tightly enough to prevent motion, but not so tight as to cut off circulation. Leave a finger or toe exposed so that you can periodically check the color and temperature to make sure that the blood supply is adequate. Swelling, a colder temperature, or a bluer color than the rest of the body are signs of inadequate circulation and call for loosening of the wrappings.

If splints are not available and cannot be improvised from materials at hand, such as battens, magazines, oars, boxes, etc., adequate splinting can be accomplished by using the rest of the person's body as a support. A few simple splinting techniques will effectively immobilize most fractures or sprains.

a. Fingers and toes

   Place a soft piece of cotton, cloth, or wad of paper between the injured digit and the ones on either side and tape them together.

b. Arm

   Any injured part from the hand to the shoulder can be immobilized by placing the arm across the chest in the "Pledge of Allegiance" position and tying it down with crossing bands so that fingers, wrist, and elbow are held tightly against the chest wall and cannot move.

c. Leg

   Hip to toe can be immobilized by placing soft cushioning material such as towels, blankets, small pillows, or rolled-up clothing between the legs, tying the legs together above and below the knees and keeping the victim flat so that the knees and hips do not bend.

Special Situations

1. Skull fracture
   See entry for Head Injury.

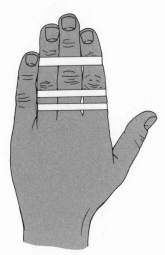

Figure 23.
Splinted finger or toe

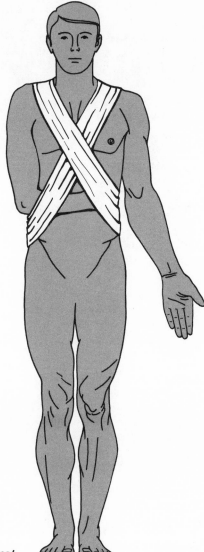

Figure 24.
Arm splinted across chest

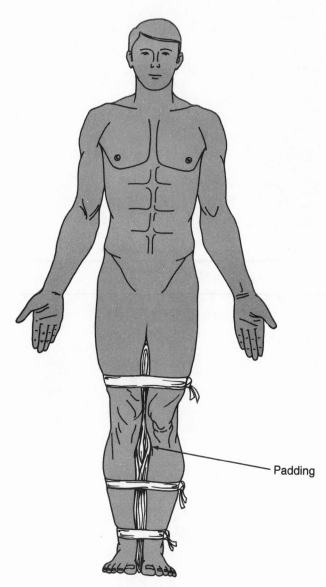

Padding

Figure 25.
Legs splinted together

2. Rib fracture

These usually don't require any special treatment beyond rest and pain medication.

3. Back and neck fractures

When you suspect one of these injuries, keep the person flat on a hard surface and as motionless as possible until you get help. Support the neck with a collar made from a rolled-up towel. If you must roll the person over onto the back do it slowly and gently. Never lift by the arms or legs.

4. Compound fractures

In addition to all the measures already described you must try to prevent infection. Wash the area thoroughly with soap and water and apply sterile dressings. Start Erythromycin, 400 mg. every six hours, and continue until you get to a physician.

Most fractures and many sprains will require definitive medical care. The best rule to follow is to leave the splints and dressings you have applied in place until you can get to a medical facility. An exception can be made for the minor sprain which is obviously well before help is available.

Head Injury: Concussion, Contusion, Skull Fracture

The brain is a soft, fragile structure floating in liquid inside a hard, bony case. Most bumps to the head don't cause serious problems because of the protection from the skull and the cushioning effect of the fluid. A hard blow, however, can cause the brain to shift and strike the inside of the skull, causing some brain injury. The range of possible injury is:

1. Concussion: swelling of the brain without tissue damage;
2. Contusion: actual injury to brain tissue;
3. Hemorrhage: bleeding into the skull cavity or brain tissue from torn blood vessels.

A fracture of the skull, unless it is depressed and pressing on the brain, is not serious in and of itself. The importance of the fracture is that it indicates a hard enough blow to the head to cause brain injury. A depressed skull fracture can usually be felt and will require surgical treatment.

Evaluation of Head Injuries

Head injury symptoms may occur immediately or show up minutes, hours, or even days after an accident. The things to watch for are:
1. Loss of consciousness
    This is the single most serious sign of brain injury. It may vary from mild drowsiness to total lack of response to sound or to pain. The deeper the stupor and the longer it lasts the more dangerous the injury and the potential for permanent brain damage or death.
2. Headache
    Persistent strong headache not relieved by aspirin is a possible warning signal of impending problems.
3. Nausea or vomiting
    Vomiting once or twice after a blow to the head is common. Persistent vomiting may indicate a more serious injury.
4. Dizziness
    Like all other brain injury symptoms, early dizziness which passes is probably not important. Persistent or late onset of dizziness may be a portent of trouble.

Specific Problem

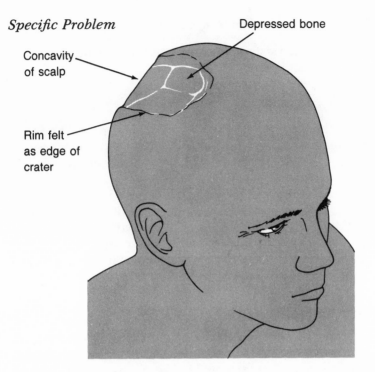

Concavity of scalp

Depressed bone

Rim felt as edge of crater

Figure 26.
Depressed skull fracture

5. Unequal pupils

These result from pressure caused by swelling of the brain with concussion and will usually correct themselves. If they persist, it may be a clue to persisting high pressure in the head, such as might occur with bleeding.

6. Blurred vision, confusion, lack of muscle coordination

Again, when these appear early and disappear soon they need not cause too much concern. When they persist or develop later, they too may be warning signals.

Treatment of Head Injuries

When signs of trauma to the brain appear, the number-one first aid measure is *rest.* The victim should stay quiet until all symptoms have subsided for several hours. It is not necessary to keep the injured person awake, but it is important to disturb him or her periodically; look for enough response to distinguish sleep from unconsciousness. Do not give pain medication or sedation stronger than aspirin. It will increase drowsiness and make the evaluation of the state of consciousness more difficult.

Coma Following Head Injury

The major danger signal of a serious head injury is decreasing state of consciousness. As long as the injured person is alert or can be aroused easily from sleep the other symptoms are of less concern. If the patient is awake enough to complain you have time to have him or her checked out when you get where you are going.

In the presence of coma or of progressively increasing lethargy, get to medical attention as soon as possible. If help is more than a short time away give Decadron injection, 4 mg. every six hours, until the victim is awake or under professional care.

Heart Attack
(coronary)

No age and neither sex is immune to the sudden, potentially devastating effects of a heart attack. The classic picture is of severe, crushing pressure and pain in the chest behind the sternum (breastplate) radiating to the left arm and accompanied by pallor, sweating, anxiety, and shortness of breath. In the presence of these events, the diagnosis is pretty obvious, even to the untrained observer. Often, however, the symptoms are more vague. The pain may be milder and more localized; the victim may feel quite well for a time. Sometimes the complaints are dismissed as severe indigestion. Denial that a heart attack could be happening is a common psychological reaction. It becomes important for the bystander to remain objective and to have some index of suspicion when chest pain persists or indigestion fails to respond to antacids, a healthy bowel movement, or a good burp.

Early treatment is the key to survival. Any suspected coronary should be considered to be an emergency, and help should be sought as quickly as possible. While waiting for professional care, these few steps may be lifesaving.

1. Demerol injection, 100 to 150 mg. every four hours, for pain and for sedation. Use the larger dose for persons over 160 pounds.
2. Oxygen.
3. Rest.
4. Reassurance: fear increases heart rate and blood pressure and, with them, risk.
5. Watch closely for signs of shock (pallor, rapid pulse, sweating, faintness). Give adrenalin (epinephrine 1-1,000) ½ ml. by injection.
6. Be prepared for CPR (cardiopulmonary resuscitation) at any time. Cardiac arrest is a constant danger. (See entry for Cardiopulmonary Resuscitation).

Heat

If, like the proverbial mad dogs and Englishmen, you must go out in the midday sun, be careful! A little warmth and sunshine can be a balm to the soul. Too much of either can be deadly. The hazards of heat and sun exposure may progress from mild discomfort to severe illness and death. Prevention is the best treatment. Avoid exposure as much as possible. Avoid excess activity. Drink plenty of liquids and eat some salty food. Avoid salt unless plenty of liquid is available. Too much salt and too little water is a dangerous combination. There are problems with absorption of many salt tablets and they are probably best avoided.

Don't ration water! Contrary to all the old teaching, the U.S. Army survival school has demonstrated that rationing water does not prolong survival time in the heat. As a matter of fact, it may be just the opposite. So drink what you have as your thirst tells you that you need it, especially in a survival situation. Your chances of survival will be greater and you will have more strength to take action to try to get rescued before it is too late. If you know beforehand that you are going to be going into a very hot environment, drink all you can before you go. It isn't only the camel that can store water.

Especially when sailing in an apparently cool breeze, the sun can be deceptive. Use protective clothing or a good sunscreen cream. There are many effective products on the market. Be sure to get a sunscreen containing para-aminobenzoic acid (PABA) rather than a tanning lotion. If you do sustain a burn, evaluate and treat it like any other burn. (See entry for Burns).

Symptoms of excess heat and sun exposure tend to build as exposure continues. If early mild warning signs are ignored the more serious problems creep insidiously up on us. The signs are:

1. Heat swelling

   This is common during the first seven to ten days in tropical climates. It is usually transient and harmless. Treatment consists of rest, elevation of the feet, and supportive dressings such as elastic bandages.

2. Exercise-induced heat collapse

   Individuals unused to hot weather may, if physically active, feel dizzy and weak or, on occasion, faint. Recovery from this unpleasant episode is almost always prompt with rest, body cooling, and lots of liquids.

3. Heat cramps

   Muscle cramping may occur secondary to salt loss. Rest, lots of liquids, and salty food will relieve this complaint.

4. Water-loss heat exhaustion

   As exposure to heat continues, loss of water through sweating may lead to more serious progression of the symptoms of faintness or cramps. If unchecked, fatigue, sweating, and giddiness may develop, to be followed by intolerable thirst, then fever, delerium, coma, and death. *Pronounced thirst* is an early important warning sign and must be heeded. Decreased urine output also shows up as an early indicator of trouble. Get cool, rest, and start drinking lots of liquids. As much as 12 pints a day may be needed to treat an average adult in the early stages and up to 8 quarts a day in more advanced heat exhaustion. With the limited water supply on most small boats the need for preventing heat exhaustion becomes apparent.

5. Salt-loss heat exhaustion

   When the body is losing salt as well as water, the symptoms become much worse much more rapidly. Thirst is generally less prominent, while headaches, severe muscle pain, nausea, vomiting, fatigue, and dizziness are more pronounced.

Treatment in this case also includes cooling, rest, and lots of liquids, but now the addition of salt is essential. A solution of 10 teaspoons of sea water to one quart of fresh water may be used.

6. Heatstroke (sunstroke)

This most lethal of all heat-induced illnesses is literally a case of being cooked. The body gradually heats up and the victim goes through some of the early stages leading to severe heat exhaustion. As a result of continued exertion and exposure, the body temperature may begin to rise while the person is still conscious, rational, and sweating. A number of factors increase individual susceptibility to heatstroke.

   a. Age: infants and older people are more prone.
   b. Fatigue.
   c. Alcohol: the habit of drinking lots of beer at hot, thirsty times may not be so smart.
   d. Inadequate fluid intake. As heating continues, sweating stops, the body temperature rises to 105° F. (40.6° C.) or more, the victim becomes confused, and, if the process is not reversed, coma and death rapidly follow.

Treatment consists of *rapid, intensive cooling!* If facilities are available, put the patient naked into a tub of ice water. A cockpit with the self-draining scuppers plugged can serve as a tub. In the absence of ice, use the coldest water at hand. Sea water is fine. Next best to an ice bath are wrapping in ice-cold wet sheets or sponging liberally with cold water in an area of free-flowing air. The immediate goal is to reduce the body temperature to 102° F. (38.9° C.) within one hour. Check the temperature every three minutes. Once that goal has been attained, stop the ice bath. Prolonging the ice bath below 102° F. may cause too great a drop in body temperature with all the attendant dangers of freezing. It is safe to continue less drastic cooling measures, such as sponge baths, since they do not cool as fast. Constant massage of the arms and legs during this time promotes circulation and speeds up cooling as the blood in the skin chills and circulates to the internal organs.

By the time the body temperature comes down to 102° F. consciousness usually will have returned, although vomiting, convulsions, and involuntary urination or bowel movement may occur along the way. As soon as possible, start oral cool liquids—as much as can be tolerated. A patient who is not conscious at that temperature or who has been unconscious for four hours or more has probably suffered some brain damage and may even die. In any event, even a survivor of heatstroke should have follow-up medical evaluation. There are many potential serious aftereffects to vital organs.

Immunizations

Vaccines are available for the prevention of many diseases. It's a good idea to maintain your immunity level against any disease to which you may be exposed for which immunization is available. For your own protection, and to meet the immunization requirements of many countries, keep an up-to-date International Certificate of Vaccination with your passport. These are to be had at all departments of health, many immigration offices, and many doctors' offices. Check with your physician or local health department regarding your immunization status.

Recommended Immunization
1. Worldwide
   These diseases are seen everywhere. In many countries immunization against them is routine during childhood and the incidence of the disease

is low. In other locales vaccination of children is not so widespread and some of the diseases still run rampant. Adults who have never received these vaccines or who have not kept their level of immunity up with the required number of boosters would be wise to get caught up.

a. Diphtheria

Three injections at one- to two-month intervals. Booster injections at intervals of one year, five years, and ten years. Total of six doses.

b. Pertussis (whooping cough)

Same as for diphtheria, but not recommended after age six years because of possible reactions unless in an epidemic area.

c. Tetanus (lockjaw)

Same initial routine as for diphtheria. After sixth dose, booster required every ten years for life. After a dirty or deep penetrating wound a booster may be advisable after five years.

d. Poliomyelitis

Triple oral polio vaccine (Trivalent Sabin) is best. Three doses two months apart. Boosters at one year and five years. Total of five doses.

e. Measles (red measles, hard measles, ten-day measles, rubeola)

One injection. Apparently good for life.

f. German measles (three-day measles, rubella)

Primarily a hazard to the fetus when contracted by a pregnant woman. One injection. Apparently good for life. Do not give to a pregnant woman or if pregnancy likely within two months.

g. Mumps

One injection. Apparently good for life.

2. Specific locales

These diseases exist regularly in certain geographic areas or may occur sporadically anywhere. Departments of health, immigration services, foreign consulates, or the World Health Organization of the United Nations can provide information about immunization requirements. When planning to visit foreign ports, check well ahead of time. Some immunizations consist of multiple doses over several week's time. Some of the diseases for which vaccines are available are:

   a. Smallpox

      This disease is almost gone from the face of the earth because of a remarkable worldwide immunization program by the World Health Organization. However, vaccination is still a requirement for entry to many countries.

   b. Cholera

   c. Yellow fever

   d. Typhoid

   e. Salmonella (paratyphoid)

   f. Plague (bubonic plague)

   g. Typhus

3. Questionable procedures

Two diseases occur for which some measure of protection is available but for which there is difference of opinion as to the need for or advisability of immunization.

   a. Hepatitis

      This is a waterborne virus infection in many parts of the world. It may also be transmitted by close personal contact with an infected individual. Gamma globulin by injection is an effective protection, but the immunity lasts only a few weeks. This makes it impractical for the long-time traveler. For a short-term visit to a high-risk area a single dose before departure may be a good idea.

   b. Tuberculosis

      A tuberculosis vaccine (BCG) is in widespread use for children in Europe. It has not been accepted as a routine procedure in the

United States. The American Academy of Pediatrics recommends this vaccine only for children with negative tuberculin skin tests who will live or travel extensively in areas where prolonged, intimate contact with tuberculosis is likely. This does not represent a high risk for the average cruising family.

Injections

The idea of giving a shot is sometimes intimidating to one who has never done it, but it isn't really very difficult. Diabetic children as young as eight years learn to measure and inject their own insulin. Some medications which might be needed in an emergency are only effective when injected. Others, which will work by mouth, may act too slowly that way or may not be usable because of decreased consciousness of the victim. The most likely needs for injectable medication at sea are:

1. Demerol for severe pain;
2. Adrenalin (Epinephrine 1 to 1000) for shock or severe allergic reactions;
3. Xylocaine for local anesthesia.

After a demonstration by a doctor or nurse and a few practice shots into a volunteer using sterile water, almost anyone should be able to give an injection with confidence. Since a long time may pass between the learning and the need to inject medications here is a step-by-step reminder of the procedure.

1. Decide which drug you want to use and the dose.
2. Check the label carefully to find the concentration of the medicine in the bottle. For example, Demerol is usually packaged with 50 mg. per 1 ml. of the

solution. (The terms *ml.* for milliliter and *cc.* for cubic centimeter are used interchangeably. They mean exactly the same thing.)

3. Figure out the amount to be injected. In the example above, 100 mg. of Demerol would require 2 ml. of solution.

4. Select the appropriate-size syringe. Use a 2-ml. syringe for amounts over 1 ml. and a 1-ml. syringe for amounts less than 1 ml. The calibrations are easier to read on the smaller syringe for measuring fractions of a ml.

5. If the drug is in an ampule, break off the tip of the ampule at the marking on the neck.

6. If the container is a rubber-stoppered bottle, wash the top with alcohol.

7. Place the needle into the container and fill the syringe to the proper line. Injecting a little air into a vacuum-sealed rubber-stoppered bottle makes it easier to withdraw the liquid.

8. Select the injection site. Safe locations are the side of the arm, the side or front of the thigh, or the upper and outer quadrant of the buttock. The larger the amount to be injected the bigger the muscle mass you want to inject it into.

9. Cleanse the injection site with alcohol.

10. Stretch the skin by pulling it between your thumb and forefinger.

11. *Jab* the needle into the skin. The slow, deliberate push may look gentler, but the quick jab penetrates the skin faster and hurts a lot less.

12. Pull gently back on the plunger of the syringe. If blood appears at the base of the syringe where the needle is attached, move the needle a bit. When no blood is seen, push the plunger in to inject the medication.

13. Pull the needle out quickly; coming out fast hurts less just like going in fast.

(M—minims—drops. Ignore this scale.)

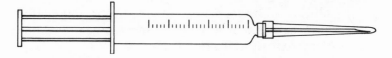

2¹/₂ cc (ml) syringe graduated in 1/10cc
increments and labelled at each ¹/₂ cc.

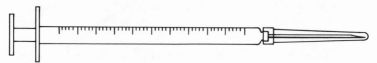

1 cc (ml) syringe graduated in 1/100cc
increments and labelled at each 1/10cc (.1 cc).

Figure 27.
1-ml. and 2-ml. syringes

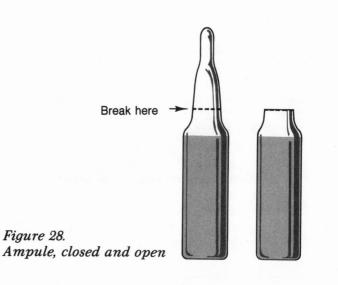

Break here →

Figure 28.
Ampule, closed and open

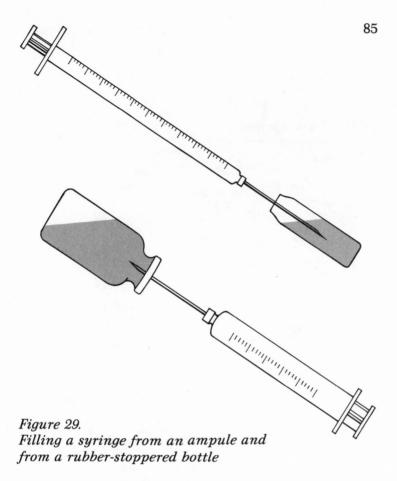

Figure 29.
Filling a syringe from an ampule and
from a rubber-stoppered bottle

Nails
(fingernails and toenails)

Perched at the tips of our fingers and toes, the nails are particularly vulnerable to injuries that are rarely serious but are always painful.

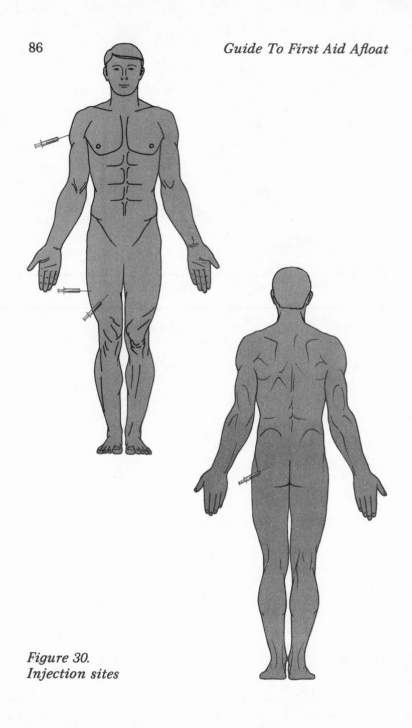

Figure 30.
Injection sites

1. Hemorrhage under the nail

   Trapped blood under pressure produces very painful throbbing. The discomfort can sometimes be relieved by soaking in ice-cold water, but frequently that will not be enough. The pain can be eliminated quickly by heating the end of a wire or paper clip in a flame until it is red hot, then pressing it firmly against the center of the nail. A small hole will burn through the nail and the blood will spurt out. The relief is immediate and no further treatment other than a Band-Aid (to keep dirt out of the hole) is usually necessary.

2. Torn nail

   A nail torn loose from its bed hurts badly. Soaking in ice water stops bleeding and eases the pain. If the nail is not completely torn away, trim the separated part with a scissors. Protect the nail bed with a Band-Aid. Apply some Vaseline or Neosporin ointment first to prevent sticking. As the nail grows more may separate, and trimming may be needed every few days.

3. Ingrown toenail

   When infected, and especially when subjected to the pressure of a shoe and the attempt to balance on a pitching, rolling deck, an ingrown toenail can be a source of much misery. A toenail may become ingrown because the nail has been cut or picked too short and a jagged corner grows into the flesh, or by the edge of the nail curling under and growing into the side of the nail bed. Prevention entails keeping the nails trimmed long and square. This eliminates ingrowing corners and permits lifting of the edge if it starts to cut the flesh. If a toenail does become ingrown, soak it in warm water two or three times a day and gently try to lift the ingrown edge with a sterilized tweezers or nail file. (Boil the instrument in water for fifteen

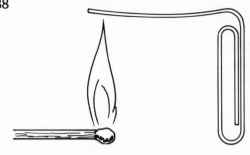

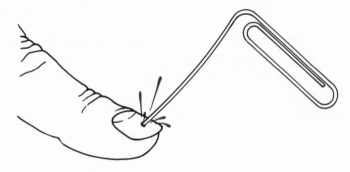

Figure 31.
Burning a hole in a fingernail

minutes.) If the area is red or if there is pus, apply Neosporin ointment after each soaking.

Pain

Pain, like fever, is a symptom of something amiss. The most obvious way to relieve the pain is to cure the cause.

Until that can be done the affected person deserves some comfort, not only for humanitarian reasons, but also because the emotional and physiologic response to pain frequently interferes with healing. There are several approaches to the reduction of pain.

1. Local

   Immobilizing sprains and fractures, applying cold compresses to injuries, covering wounds, and changing body position will frequently help to ease pain.

2. Reassurance

   Anxiety increases the level of pain and decreases the tolerance to it. Tender loving care is a great sedative.

3. Specific pain medication

   a. Mild

   Aspirin or acetaminophen (Tylenol, Datril, Tempra, Phenaphen) are effective treatment for mild pain. Follow dosage directions on the label. *A larger than recommended dose does not usually increase the pain relief, but always increases the risk of toxic side effects.* There are many combinations available, such as Anacin, Empirin, Alka-Seltzer and a host of others. Basically, they all depend on the same pain relievers and are probably no more effective than aspirin or acetaminophen alone.

   b. Intermediate

   Codeine is probably the most commonly used pain medication when milder drugs don't work. Unfortunately, many people cannot tolerate codeine and develop nausea or headaches. Effective substitutes are Darvon, Percodan, or Talwin.

   All of these drugs are classified either as narcotics or dangerous drugs and require prescriptions. The physician who writes the prescription should know the age and weight of each potential user of the medication and provide written dose instructions for each individual.

c. Strong

For very severe pain, such as that caused by large burns, fractures, heart attacks, and other major medical problems, only very potent narcotic drugs like morphine or Demerol will be effective. These are dangerous, difficult to obtain, and require injection. The conditions which call for their use are serious, urgent, and require immediate medical attention. For the average boater, who remains within reasonable distance of emergency care, it is probably wisest to leave the administration of such drugs to the professional. For the transoceanic sailor the problem is different. With many days and many miles between you and help it may be essential to be prepared to offer relief for intolerable pain. Again, whoever provides the prescription should provide dosage recommendations.

A Few Words of Warning!

We have been talking about the use of narcotic drugs. Their use for any but medical purposes is illegal everywhere in the world. In many places possession of these drugs by any but licensed doctors or hospitals is forbidden. Penalties for misuse, importation, and exportation are very severe. To keep out of trouble follow a few basic rules.

1. Carry no more than reasonable, prudent people would recognize as legitimate to cover possible emergencies.
2. Keep a photostatic copy of the prescription and, if possible, a letter from the prescribing physician explaining the reason for the prescription.
3. Check with the consulates of the places you plan to visit. Tell them what you plan to carry and ask

what the policy is in their country. If you get approval, get it in writing. If there is any doubt, leave the stuff behind.

4. *Always* declare the drugs at customs entering or leaving a country. If you do, the likelihood is that the officials will let you keep it or, at worst, will impound it. Failure to declare is a sure ticket to the lockup if the drugs are discovered.

Poisoning

Poisoning may be accidental or deliberate. It may result from the intake of poisonous food, chemicals, medicines, or nonmedicinal drugs. Some poisons may act by absorption through the skin or by inhalation. Symptoms produced by different types of poisons are so varied, treatment is so difficult and nonspecific, and so many poisons are deadly that the best treatment is prevention. Know what you are eating and drinking, know what you are using. Read labels. Follow instructions carefully.

Pay special attention to children! Little ones are naturally curious creatures. There is almost nothing, regardless of taste or smell, that some youngster won't try. On a boat, even more than on land, deadly temptations may be hard to hide. The fuel supply, the cleaning materials, and the medical kit are all potential sources of accidental death. Keep all poisonous materials secured out of the reach of tiny hands and mouths!

Sources of Poison

1. Food
   a. Toxic animals and plants
      Survival schools teach that the number of poisonous animals and plants is so small that if you are in danger of starving to death you should eat anything that doesn't eat you first. Under normal

conditions we can afford to be a little more selective. The wild mushroom, the pufferfish, the oleander berry, and the manchineel apple are probably well known to most cruisers to be deadly, but many other attractive-looking killers may be less familiar. Local knowledge can introduce you to many new taste treats and at the same time protect you from dangers. Cruising guides are often good sources.

b. Botulism

This deadly disease is caused by a poison produced by bacteria in improperly canned foods. Very careful attention to sanitary and sterile procedures is the only prevention. A specific antitoxin is the only cure. Death is agonizing and rapid. If you don't know how something was preserved, avoid it. If you have doubts about something you prepared yourself, get rid of it.

c. "Food poisoning"

This incorrect name is commonly applied to vomiting and diarrhea caused by infected or spoiled food. Prevention consists of careful washing of food and dishes, proper cooking, boiling of suspect water, and proper food storage to prevent spoiling. Treatment is discussed in the entries for Vomiting and Diarrhea.

2. Chemicals

Most toxic substances have warning labels regarding eating, drinking, skin contact, or breathing vapors. Cleansers, insecticides, fuels, and solvents are all potential poisons. Read labels carefully. If there is no label, assume that any chemical may be deadly and handle with care. Use gloves, don't use it near food, and keep the working area well ventilated.

3. Medications

The most beneficial medicine can turn into a killer when used improperly. Follow dosage instructions with care. Even so common a friend as aspirin will turn on us and destroy us if we take too much. A good general rule to remember is that if recommended doses don't do the job, increased doses usually do not increase the benefits but always increase the risks.

4. Nonmedicinal drugs

What a waste to "OD" looking for a kick or an escape. Cruising the seas and exploring new places should be such a trip in itself that no drug-induced high should be necessary. A bad "trip" is so often a one way ticket to hell that gambling with drugs is just plain stupid!

Immediate First Aid for Poisoning

1. Separate the person from the poison as fast as possible.

    a. Skin contact

    Remove clothing and wash skin thoroughly.

    b. Inhalation

    Get away from the fumes and into the fresh air.

    c. Swallowing

    Induce vomiting.

    Petroleum products (gasoline, kerosene, and certain solvents) should *not* be vomited. For other poisons use syrup of Ipecac:

    Children under 1 year—1 to 2 teaspoons. Over 2 years—3 teaspoons.

    Repeat in twenty minutes if vomiting has not occurred.

    If Ipecac is not available, a strong salt solution will frequently induce vomiting. Even a finger down the throat sometimes works.

2. After vomiting stops—or, in the case of petroleum products, immediately—give milk if available, mineral oil, or absorbent food such as bread. They may help to bind the poison and reduce the absorption into the system of any which was not vomited.

Specific Treatment for Poisoning

1. Treat any symptoms which develop using the techniques described in the entries dealing with the specific problems, such as pain, vomiting, diarrhea, etc. Sadly, the effects of many poisons are beyond the limits of first aid care.
2. Call for medical advice whenever possible. The variety of poisons and the symptoms they can produce, as well as possible antidotes and specific treatment, is too vast for a volume such as this.
3. Check labels. Many packages containing poisonous substances will carry instructions for treatment.
4. Universal antidote. Would it were so, but, unfortunately, the existence of a single antidote against all poisons remains an elusive myth.

Rabies
(hydrophobia)

This horrible, always fatal disease occurs everywhere. It has been recorded in history as early as 800 B.C. The infecting virus is carried in the saliva of diseased animals. Dogs, cats, squirrels, skunks, wolves, and all sorts of rodents, including bats, may be sources of infection. The virus is transmitted by contact between the infected saliva and broken skin. The animal carrying the disease does not necesarily behave like the traditional "mad dog," so playing with strange stray animals is not safe. If bitten, follow these steps:

1. Don't panic!
   The incubation period for rabies is very long. Rabies is a brain disease. The virus travels along nerves to the brain, not through the blood stream, so the further the bite is from the head the more time you

have. Even in bites of the head and neck there are several days in which to act.

2. Try to kill or capture the animal.
   If possible, do not damage the head. By examining the brain, a pathologist can tell whether or not the animal had rabies.

3. Cleanse the wound thoroughly with soap and water and apply Betadine or alcohol. It won't prevent rabies, but will help to prevent other infections which may follow animal bites.

4. Get to the nearest health facility as soon as possible, with or without the animal. If the creature has rabies, or cannot be found, you will need to take a series of injections of antirabies vaccine. This is an unpleasant but fortunately very effective preventive measure. And the newer vaccines are neither as painful nor as toxic as were the older ones.

Respiratory Infections (colds, flu, sore throat, bronchitis, pneumonia)

Most respiratory infections, especially in adults, are caused by viruses and are self-limited. The only treatment needed is rest, lots of liquids, and the relief of symptoms. Aspirin for fever or pain, decongestants, cough medicines, etc., all can make you feel better while the infection cures itself. Everyone has a favorite "cold remedy." There is little difference between them, so use what makes you feel better. One caution: some combinations contain aspirin. Check labels carefully so that you don't take additional aspirin at the same time and risk an overdose.

Under certain conditions, if a medical diagnosis is not obtainable, it may be wise to treat with antibiotics. The rationale for making that decision is that treating a virus unnecessarily may be less risky than not treating a more serious bacterial infection.

Indications for Antibiotic Treatment

1. Cough, sore throat, fever, swollen glands persist more than one or two days.
2. Fever is getting higher and patient is getting sicker.
3. Fever develops after symptoms have been present for several days without fever.

Choice of Antibiotic

1. Erythromycin, 400 mg. every six hours, for adults. For children, use 5 mg. per pound of body weight every six hours.
2. If there is no improvement after forty-eight hours, switch to ampicillin, 500 mg. every six hours. For children use 10 mg. per pound of body weight every six hours.

It is very important to continue treatment, with whichever medication is helping for ten days, even though symptoms may be gone. Stopping too soon may lead to relapses, which can be worse than the original disease, especially if a half-killed colony of bacteria has had a chance to develop immunity to the antibiotic.

Seasickness
(Is it all in your head?)

As a matter of fact, it probably is, if not all in your head, at least a good part there, in a little bony labyrinth in your ear. When the fluid in that labyrinth gets jiggled about, it activates nerve endings which trigger nausea, dizziness, and some of the other terrible symptoms of mal de mer. Add fatigue, anxiety, and hunger, and there isn't one of us who might not suffer from this affliction at one time or another. For reasons which are not fully understood, some people are more susceptible than others.

1. Try not to get overtired; when you are off watch, rest.
2. Don't get too hungry; an empty stomach and low blood sugar apparently increase the chances of getting sick.
3. If you are feeling uneasy, keep busy; activity seems to divert the onset of symptoms.
4. If you are feeling queasy stay on deck if possible; confined spaces usually make matters worse. If you must be below, lie down and close your eyes.
5. Take an appropriate preventive medication. The key word is "preventive"; once you are sick no medicine seems to help. Whatever you use, take it at least an hour before going to sea and repeat at the prescribed intervals. Most sailors get their "sea legs" eventually, so on a long passage skip a dose after a day or two to see if you still need it.
6. Seasick "remedies"

    a. Dramamine or Marezine

    These are available without prescription and are effective for many people. Unfortunately, they don't work for everyone and they can cause excessive drowsiness.

    b. Triptone

    This nonprescription item contains 0.25 mg. of scopolamine, which is one of the drugs on the list of the National Aeronautics and Space Administration's list of apparently effective drugs for preventing motion sickness.

    c. Bucladin

    Some years ago this product was on the market as a tablet with five ingredients. For the intractable seasick-prone sailor, it proved to be an almost infallible preventive. Literally dozens of my sailing companions, as well as I, find it indispensable. Unfortunately, the new tablet does not seem to have the beneficial effect of the previous one. However, it is possible to have the ingredients compounded into a capsule and to reproduce the original formula. A prescription is required and many pharmacists are unwilling to spend the time needed to make the capsules. If you are truly seasick-prone, you may find it worth your while to search for someone who will do the job. The formula can be found in the *Physicians' Desk Reference,* 1975 edition. It is as follows:

Buclizine HC1 . . . . . 50/0 mg.
Pyridoxine HC1 . . . . 10/0 mg.
Scopolamine HBr. . . 0/2 mg.
Atropine SO_4 . . . . . . 0/05 mg.
Hyoscamine SO_4 . . . 0/05 mg.

The dose is one every six hours. Ask your doctor. If there is no contraindication to your taking any of the ingredients, try it.

Shock
(the silent killer)

What is it, this quiet assassin that creeps up on us when our attention is elsewhere and destroys the life we are trying to save? Shock is "a state of profound depression of the vital processes of the body characterized by pallor, rapid but weak pulse, rapid and shallow respiration, restlessness, anxiety or mental dullness, and sometimes nausea or vomiting. The total blood volume is reduced. The blood pressure is low and the temperature subnormal. Shock occurs as a result of extensive wounds, hemorrhage, crushing injuries, blows inflicting extreme pain, prolonged surgical operation, etc., and is designated 'primary' or 'secondary' according as symptoms supervene immediately after the injury or some hours later."*

Sound terrible? It is, and for purposes of first aid there is little or nothing you can do to treat it. Treatment requires replacement of blood volume with appropriate intravenous fluids, such as blood, plasma, or synthetic "blood expanders," oxygen, and other measures only available in a hospital.

You can, however, do a great deal to prevent shock from developing. Each of the steps which you take as you move through the Emergency Game Plan, from the restoration of heartbeat and breathing to the relief of pain and fear, is a vital preventive measure against shock.

Sometimes, when it appears that shock is imminent (victim is sweating, pale, and feeling faint) an injection of Adrenalin (Epinephrine 1 to 1000) (½ ml.) may reverse the process.

If, despite all your efforts, shock does develop, unless definitive medical care is close at hand you may have reached one of the limits of your ability to help.

Skin

The skin is subject to many insults. Allergies, infections, and many internal diseases can produce an outbreak on the skin. Telling the different eruptions apart is often a challenge even to an experienced eye. Keeping the skin clean and dry, using powder after cleansing, and avoiding too much sun will help avoid many skin problems on a boat.

*Webster's New International Dictionary, Second Edition.

Allergic Rashes

Redness with itching, blotches, scaliness, or hives are the usual signs of skin allergy. Treatment aims at relief of discomfort and removal of the offending substance if it can be identified.

1. Avoid soap and other irritants. Keep clean by gentle rinsing with cool water.
2. Keep raw, moist surfaces covered.
3. Relieve itching.

> a. A solution of baking soda (1 tablespoon to 8 ounces of water) as a compress is helpful.
>
> b. Chlor-Trimeton, 4 mg. every four hours (may cause drowsiness), brings relief.

Skin Infections

1. Bacterial infections (boils, impetigo, cellulitis)
   Redness with pain rather than itching, the presence of pus or a greasy crust are the hallmarks of these skin lesions. Treatment is directed at eradication of the bacteria.

   > a. Local warm compresses for fifteen to twenty minutes several times a day.
   >
   > b. Neosporin ointment to the sores after each compress.
   >
   > c. For large or spreading infections give Erythromycin, 400 mg. every six hours. Continue for ten days even if the eruption has healed. If there is no improvement in forty-eight hours switch to ampicillin, 500 mg. every six hours.

2. Virus infections (herpes, cold sores, shingles)
   These may appear as a localized eruption or cover an extensive area paralleling a nerve root. There is generally both pain and itching. The lesion starts as a small blister which gradually dries to form a scab. Frequently, nearby glands are swollen and sore. There may be slight oozing of clear

serum, but there is no pus. The small local variety (herpes simplex, cold sore) will take one to two weeks from the first discomfort until the scab falls off. The more extensive form (herpes zoster, shingles) is caused by a different virus and may persist for as long as six weeks. Local treatment for either type of herpes is very unsatisfactory and can sometimes be harmful. Keep the sores clean and dry. Use whatever pain medication is necessary for comfort.

3. Fungus infections (athlete's foot, jock itch, etc.)
   Fungus loves to grow in warm, moist places. The feet, the armpits, and the crotch are favorite sites for these miserable rashes. Itching, redness, and scaling are the most prominent features. The location and a shiny glistening appearance to the redness help to differentiate these from allergic rashes.
   Frequent washing, frequent changes of clothes, and the use of Desenex powder in shoes several times a day plus the application of Desenex ointment or Lotrimin cream to the affected areas will usually clear these up. It takes a long time, and even after the skin has cleared the fungus may remain, so continue the treatment for several days after you think the rash is gone.

Rashes which do not fall into one of the above categories or which do not clear with the recommended treatment may be indicators of more serious illness and should be evaluated by a doctor. Until medical help is available, avoid irritants and use pain medication or antihistamine (Chlor-Trimeton, 4 mg. every four hours) as needed to relieve pain or itching and leave the rash alone.

Snake Bite

On the land and in the sea there are snakes whose fangs carry death. Species vary from place to place and the venom varies from species to species. When a snake bites, first aid treatment is required urgently. A good snake bite kit puts the things you need right at hand. With no kit available improvise with whatever you have.

1. Restrict the circulation of venom from the bite to the body. Apply a tourniquet close to the bite on the side nearest to the heart. If the bite is on the trunk, rather than on an arm or a leg, a tight binder around the body just above the bite may help.
2. Cut across the bite marks.
3. Apply suction.
   The suction cup supplied with the snake bite kit is best. Suction can be applied by mouth, but there is some risk of absorbing venom through a crack in the lip or the lining of the mouth.
4. Get medical care *fast!*
   Only specific antivenin is truly lifesaving. The snake, dead or alive, or an accurate description is a big help in identifying the correct antivenin.

Stings
(venomous marine animals)

On the land there are many insects whose stings can cause unpleasant reactions (see the entry for Allergies). Distributed widely through the oceans of the world are a large number of creatures that sting. They are found more often in the warmer waters and among the reefs and lagoons which are the favored playgrounds of the cruising sailor. Unlike the bee, the wasp, and the ant, which most of us instinctively avoid, these beings, neither fish nor mammal, are usually brilliant in color, exotic in shape, and graceful in motion, inviting an intimacy which at best can cause discomfort and at worst almost instant death. Hidden on the tentacles of the jellyfish, sea anemone, Portugese man-of-war (bluebottle), hydroid (those plumelike tufts that grow on rocks and pilings), sea wasp, and sea nettle are tiny stinging cells waiting to inject their poison into the unwary. Many forms of coral, too, bear cells as deadly as poison darts. Very little is known about the nature of the venom carried by these Hydrozoans, and treatment is less than satisfactory. The best rule is to avoid physical contact with them, alive or dead. The stinging cells, even in a seemingly dead animal, can be activated by touch. Swimming among the reefs without protective covering, walking barefoot, and reaching bare-handed into dark places should be avoided.

The stinging cell (nematocyst) comes in many shapes, but consists basically of a toxin-filled capsule, a tube, and a pointed tip. When touched the tube darts out to sting and the capsule contracts to inject the poison. The reaction produced depends on the species of animal, the part of the body stung, and the individual susceptibility of the victim. Symptoms may be as varied as local redness, hives, peeling, hemorrhage, chills, fever, diarrhea, severe shooting pains, joint pains, swollen glands, headache, nausea, vomiting, fainting, sneezing, abdominal pain, blueness, shock, and death.

Treatment of the stings from these killers is directed at three main goals.

1. Eliminate toxic effects
   a. Remove tentacles *fast!*

They may be too small to see. Remove clothes, and rub the skin vigorously with *dry* sand, cloth, paper towels, etc.

b. For coral cuts, scrub the area thoroughly, remove all visible particles with a knife or tweezers, and apply a strong antiseptic, such as Betadine.

c. Apply tourniquets.

If the sting is on an arm or leg, place the tourniquet between the sting and the heart, elevate the extremity and keep it at rest.

d. Apply alcohol, suntan lotion, Vaseline, or oil to the area. These all inhibit toxic activity.

e. If a local reaction appears, apply cortisone cream. If none is available, try sugar, soap, vinegar, lemon juice, ammonia solution, or baking soda.

f. Antihistamine by mouth.

Chlor-Trimeton, 4 mg. every four hours.

2. Control pain

The pain can be excruciating. Demerol, 100 to 150 mg. by injection, may be necessary. Use the larger dose for persons over 160 pounds. For milder pain use milder remedies (see the entry for Pain).

3. Sustain life

a. At the first sign of shock (pallor, sweating, faintness) give adrenalin (epinephrine 1 to 1000) ½ ml. by injection.

b. Be prepared for CPR (see entry for Cardiopulmonary Resuscitation).

c. Get medical help if possible. In addition to life-saving equipment, some medical facilities have the specific antivenin, which is rare but does exist for a few species.

Tropical Diseases

Tropical lands can assault the body with bizarre and often deadly diseases even as they excite the imagination with exotic sights and sounds. Strange-sounding names, like Dengue fever, schistosomiasis, filariasis, and Amebiasis, join the list of dangers along with the more familiar malaria, cholera, plague, yellow fever, typhus, and typhoid. The enemy may be a bacteria, a parasite, or a worm. Transmission of the disease may be through water, food, soil, or any number of biting animals or insects. Symptoms are many and varied and usually severe. Incubation periods range from days to weeks. Treatment is specific for each disease but, for some, not always effective.

Prevention of Tropical Disease

1. Avoid insect bites.
   a. Screen hatches and ports.
   b. Use netting over bunks.
   c. Use insect repellents.
   d. Wear protective clothing.
   e. Vitamin B1, 50 mg. daily by mouth, may produce an insect-repelling body odor.
2. Keep bugs and rodents off the boat.
   a. Spray regularly with insecticide. Check the label carefully for toxic precautions.
   b. Don't bring paper bags or cartons from local markets aboard. They frequently harbor eggs of insects, especially roaches, which can hatch into very unpleasant and disease-bearing little beasts.
   c. Place large enough guards on dock lines to prevent rodents from climbing aboard.
3. Purify water.
   Boil water for twenty minutes or use a commercial water purifier.

4. Cook food well.
5. Peel fruits and vegetables.
6. Don't walk barefoot.
7. Don't pet animals.
8. Don't swim in rivers or lakes in areas where these diseases are prevalent.
9. Use immunizing procedures when available (see the entry for Immunizations).
10. For regions where malaria is a major problem, Chloroquine (Aralen phosphate) is an effective preventive. It is also potentially very toxic. Its use should be carefully evaluated with the help of the doctor who prescribes it.

Diagnosis of Tropical Diseases

1. Unusual or prolonged symptoms of any kind during or within a few weeks after a visit to a tropical country should be suspect.
2. Specific laboratory tests are needed to identify most of these illnesses. See a doctor as soon as possible. Be sure to tell him where you have been.

Treatment of Tropical Diseases

Until a diagnosis has been made you can only treat symptoms such as fever, pain, diarrhea, or vomiting in a nonspecific way. Each of these is discussed in its own entry.

Urinary System

The kidneys and bladder are vulnerable to two problems, especially in hot climates, where fluid intake is inadequate and urine becomes concentrated.

1. Kidney stones

   More common in men and frequently smaller than a pea, these little devils can be the cause of one of the worst pains known. Excruciating, incapacitating pain may originate in the lower back, radiate around the abdomen, and down to the groin. It may be accompanied by a feeling of pressure over the bladder and a frequent, urgent need to urinate. Sometimes there is bright red blood in the urine. The pain may vary with the size of the stone. As the stone migrates from the kidney to the bladder the discomfort moves downward. Most stones eventually pass spontaneously in the urine. The time for passage may be hours, days, or weeks. Pain will often come and go with long intervals of comfort.

   Treatment consists of drinking lots of liquids and using the strongest necessary pain medication (see entry for Pain). If the pain persists or the stone does not pass, get medical attention. Some stones are too big to go through the narrow passages. They can block the kidney and, if not surgically removed, may cause permanent kidney damage.

2. Urinary infections

   More common in women, the symptoms of infection may be similar to those of stones, but are usually less severe. There may be fever; its presence is a good clue to infection, but its absence does not eliminate the possibility.

   Treatment has two major goals.

   a. Relief of symptoms

      Drinking lots of liquids helps to flush out infection and to dilute the urine so that it causes less burning.

      Pyridium, 200 mg. three times a day after meals, helps to relieve pain, burning, and urgency and frequency of urination. It does not treat the infection. The reddish tinge to the urine which frequently goes with the use of Pyridium is no cause for concern.

b. Elimination of infection

If the symptoms are well controlled and the individual is not very sick and has no fever, a delay of a week or ten days in making a diagnosis and starting treatment is safe. If, however, the symptoms persist, the patient is feeling sick or has fever, or if medical attention is more than a week or ten days away, antibiotic treatment should be started. First choice would be Gantrisin, 500-mg. tablets. Give four tablets to start, then two tablets every four hours (be sure to ask about allergy to sulfa drugs). If Gantrisin is not available, or if there is a possibility of sulfa allergy, use ampicillin, 500 mg. every eight hours, or Tetracycline 250 mg. every 6 hours.

Treatment with either of these medications should be continued for two weeks. Follow-up examination of the urine is essential. Symptoms may be gone but the infection not be completely eradicated, and recurrences with serious chronic kidney disease could develop.

Venereal Diseases

After a long sea voyage the charm of a port of call often includes more than waving palms, blue lagoons, and exotic food and drink. For the lonely sailor who travels without a mate the satisfying of certain romantic urges sometimes carries a high price tag. Alas, the cost may be in health rather than in currency. The gentleman and the lady mariner are equally susceptible to the lure of amour and, unfortunately, to the risk of infection.

1. Gonorrhea (clap)

    The subject of innumerable not-so-funny jokes, this always uncomfortable, sometimes damaging disease is no laughing matter. It can lead to permanent impairment of the urinary and reproductive systems, as well as produce serious generalized body illness. The most common early symptoms, usually appearing within two to seven days after intercourse, are burning urination, a discharge of pus from the penis or vagina, and, occasionally but not often, a fever. Women may skip the early complaints only to find themselves with serious illness at a later time. Periodic gynecologic examination may help to identify an infection and prevent future complications.

    If symptoms do develop after a recent exposure, early medical attention is the wisest course. When such care is more than a week away it is a good idea to start treatment. There are a number of alternatives. Two choices which would fit with the contents of a well-equipped cruising medical kit would be:

    a. Tetracycline, 500-mg. tablets: three tablets to start, then one tablet every six hours for one week.

    b. Ampicillin, 500-mg. tablets: seven tablets as a single dose.

    Since there are treatment failures with any medication, be sure to see a doctor for follow-up evaluation as soon as possible.

2. Syphilis (lues)

    A destroyer of bodies and of minds, this insidious disease can easily be missed until it is far advanced. The earliest sign is frequently the chancre, a *painless* ulcer appearing at the point of contact several days to several weeks after exposure. Untreated, the chancre spontaneously heals while the disease spreads into the body and causes destruction not only to the patient, but in the case of infected women to children as yet unconceived. In the absence of pain the sore under the foreskin of an uncircumcized male or within the vagina of a female may come and go unnoticed. In such cases the only diagnostic tool available is a blood test, which becomes positive six weeks or longer after the original contact. Periodic blood tests are a good idea for those who have sexual contact with unknown partners.

Anyone developing a suspicious sore after sexual contact should get medical attention as soon as possible. Remember that the chancre develops at the point of sexual contact; fingers and mouths are not immune. Syphilis is a complex disease whose diagnosis and treatment are beyond the limits of this volume.

Vomiting

Vomiting does not necessarily indicate a stomach disorder. It may be a reflex response to any illness, injury, or emotional upset. It is an unpleasant symptom at best. If it persists it may not only interfere with attempts to treat the underlying problem, but, like prolonged diarrhea, may lead to dehydration. Since the vomiting patient has difficulty retaining oral medication, there are a number of rectal suppositories available containing drugs aimed at the control of vomiting. They all require prescription and have some potential undesirable side effects. A reasonably effective, reasonably safe choice is Tigan. The dose is one 200-mg. suppository inserted into the rectum every four hours for adults. For children there is a 100-mg. suppository, or the 200-mg. suppository can be cut in half. Children's doses are:

Under 30 pounds: 100 mg. every eight hours.

30 to 90 pounds: 100 mg. every six hours.

Continue until there has been no vomiting for eight to twelve hours. As soon as vomiting is under control start oral liquids. If the vomiting has been prolonged and frequent, a solution of 10 teaspoons of sea water dissolved in one full quart of fresh water may be used to avoid dehydration.

Section III
The Medical Kit

Planning the Medical Kit

1. Contents

   Physical space, budgetary considerations, and personal attitudes all impose limits on the amount and variety of medical supplies which can be carried on a small vessel. The contents to be listed in the Suggested Medical Kit presuppose an extended voyage with long-time periods away from medical care and a willingness to assume certain risks and responsibilities in a medical crisis. Each boat owner will need to make a selection based on a number of factors which will influence the final decisions.

   a. What to carry

   Where are you going? What are the potential health problems? How far will medical help be? Geography, as well as the age, sex, and physical status of crew members will be elements governing the choices to be made.

   b. How much to carry

   A by-guess and by-gosh decision at best, the answer depends on the number of crew members, the dosage of certain medications, and an estimate of the likelihood of needing any given item.

2. Organization of the kit

   A medical kit is useless if it is not readily accessible or if it is hard to find specific items that you need in a hurry. There are several ways to make things easy to find. One good method is to package together all items which fit a particular category. Label each package with the category and label each item in the package with its individual name and dose if it is a medicine.

3. Cautions
    a. Read labels carefully.
    b. Follow dosage instructions accurately.
    c. Always ask about allergies before giving any medication.

Suggested Medical Kit

Injectables

1. Decadron solution, 4 mg. per ml.*
2. Adrenalin (epinephrine 1 to 1000).*
3. Demerol, 4 mg. per ml.*
4. Sterile 2-ml. syringes with 23-gauge needles.*
5. Sterile 1-ml. syringes with 25-gauge needles.*

Injuries

1. Assorted sizes of Band-Aids.
2. Sterile packages of 2×2-inch and 4×4-inch sterile gauze pads.
3. Adhesive tape.
4. Sterile roller gauze of the self-clinging type.
5. Cotton balls.
6. Q-tips.
7. Box of assorted finger splints.
8. Wrist splints, right-handed and left-handed.
9. Betadine solution.
10. Package of Steri-Strips.
11. Package of sterile Vaseline gauze.
12. Suture set, packaged and sterile. Needle holder, thumb forceps, scissors.
13. Sterile packages of #4-0 silk suture material on swedged-on needles.
14. 1% Xylocaine local anesthetic solution*

Seasickness

1. Dramamine.
2. Marezine.
3. Triptone.
4. Bucladin.*

*Requires a prescription.

Pain (Oral Medications)

1. Aspirin, 5-grain tablets or capsules.
2. Acetaminophen (Tylenol, Datril, Phenaphen, Tempra), 5-grain tablets or capsules.
3. Empirin Compound with Codeine #3.*
4. Acetaminophen with Codeine #3.*
5. Pyridium, 100-mg. tablets.*

Infection

1. Erythromycin, 400-mg.* or capsules
2. Gantrisin, 500-mg. tablets.*
3. Ampicillin, 500-mg. tablets.*
4. Tetracycline, 250-mg.* or capsules
5. Nafcillin, 500-mg. tablets.*
6. Chloroquine tablets (for malaria only).*

Allergies

Chlor-Trimeton, 4-mg. tablets.

Digestive System

1. Lomotil tablets (syrup for children).*
2. Colace tablets (syrup for children).
3. Fleet enema (pediatric strength for children).
4. Glycerin suppositories.
5. Enema bag or rectal bulb syringe.
6. Pepto-Bismol.
7. Tigan, 200-mg. suppositories.*

Respiratory System

1. Cough medicine. Any mild nonprescription medication.
2. Phenergan Expectorant with Codeine.*

*Requires a prescription.

3. Nose drops or nasal spray. Any brand.
4. Antihistamine/decongestant ("cold remedy"). Any brand which does not contain aspirin.

Poisoning

Syrup of Ipecac.

Sedation

Valium, 5-mg. tablets.*

Local Applications (eyes, ears, skin)

1. Visine eye drops.
2. 10% Sulamyd ophthalmic solution.*
3. Cortisporin otic solution.*
4. Sun filter cream with Para-aminobenzoic acid (PABA).
5. Vaseline.
6. Desenex ointment and powder.
7. Neosporin ointment.
8. Rubbing alcohol.
9. Hydrocortisone cream or lotion.*
10. Lotrimin cream.*

Miscellaneous Equipment

1. Oxygen tank and mask.
2. Snake bite kit.

*Requires a prescription.